TWO WEEKS TO PACES
Practical Assessment
of Clinical Examination Skills

TWO WEEKS TO PACES
Practical Assessment of Clinical Examination Skills

Dr. H. Haboubi
MBBS, BSc(Hons), PhD, FRCP(UK),
Consultant Gastroenterologist & General Physician
University Hospital Llandough, Cardiff, Wales, UK

Dr. N. Ali
MBBS, MRCP (UK), MRCGP (UK), MSc, MD
GP Registrar, West Midlands Deanery
Honorary Cardiology Teaching Fellow SPR
Warwick Hospital, South Warwickshire NHS Trust, UK

Dr. A. Al-Ansari
MBBS, BA, MRCP (UK)
Specialist Registrar in Neurology
Wales Deanery, UK

World Scientific

NEW JERSEY · LONDON · SINGAPORE · BEIJING · SHANGHAI · HONG KONG · TAIPEI · CHENNAI · TOKYO

Published by

World Scientific Publishing Co. Pte. Ltd.
5 Toh Tuck Link, Singapore 596224
USA office: 27 Warren Street, Suite 401-402, Hackensack, NJ 07601
UK office: 57 Shelton Street, Covent Garden, London WC2H 9HE

British Library Cataloguing-in-Publication Data
A catalogue record for this book is available from the British Library.

TWO WEEKS TO PACES
Practical Assessment of Clinical Examination Skills

Copyright © 2021 by World Scientific Publishing Co. Pte. Ltd.

All rights reserved. This book, or parts thereof, may not be reproduced in any form or by any means, electronic or mechanical, including photocopying, recording or any information storage and retrieval system now known or to be invented, without written permission from the publisher.

For photocopying of material in this volume, please pay a copying fee through the Copyright Clearance Center, Inc., 222 Rosewood Drive, Danvers, MA 01923, USA. In this case permission to photocopy is not required from the publisher.

ISBN 978-981-121-505-6 (paperback)
ISBN 978-981-121-506-3 (ebook for institutions)
ISBN 978-981-121-507-0 (ebook for individuals)

For any available supplementary material, please visit
https://www.worldscientific.com/worldscibooks/10.1142/11686#t=suppl

Printed in Singapore

TWO WEEKS TO PACES

Dr. H. Haboubi
MBBS, BSc (Hons), PhD, FRCP (UK)
Consultant Gastroenterologist & General Physician
University Hospital Llandough, Cardiff, Wales

Dr. N. Ali
MBBS, MRCP (UK), MRCGP (UK), MSc, MD
GP Registrar, West Midlands Deanery
Honorary Cardiology Teaching Fellow SPR
Warwick Hospital, South Warwickshire NHS Trust

Dr A. Al-Ansari
MBBS, BA, MRCP (UK)
Specialist Registrar in Neurology
Wales Deanery

CONTENTS

Preface — xi
About the Authors — xv
Acknowledgement — xvii

Communication Encounters (Stations 1A & 4A) — 1

Introduction — 2
Ethics — 2
Capacity — 3
Witholding/Withdrawing Life Proloning Treatment — 5
Communication — 7
Case 1: Breaking Bad News — 9
Case 2: The Angry Relative/Complaints — 12
Case 3: Fitness To Drive — 14
Case 4: Industrial Injury Benefits — 17
Case 5: Negligence — 19
Case 6: Discussing Organ Donation — 21
Case 7: Gillick Competence — 23
Case 8: Life Insurance And Genetic Disorders — 24

Clinical Consultations (Stations 2 & 5) — 27

Introduction — 28
Case 1: Headache — 34
Case 2: Pleuritic Chest Pain — 36
Case 3: Alteration of Bowel Habits — 40
Case 4: Syncope — 43
Case 5: Deranged Liver Function Tests — 47
   Supplementary Case: Wilson's Disease — 49
Case 6: Occupational Asthma — 50
Connective Tissue Disorders & Vasculitides — The 2W2P Method — 53
Case 7: Deforming Arthritis Involving Small Hand Joints — 57
   7A — Rheumatoid Arthritis — 57
   7B — Psoriatic Arthritis — 63
   A Brief Review of Agents Used In RA & PsA For PACES — 68
Case 8: Ankylosing Spondylosis — The Archetypical Seronegative Spondarthritis — 70

Case 9: Systemic Connective Tissue Disorders 73
    9A — Systemic Sclerosis 73
    9B — Systemic Lupus Erythematosus 78
Endocrine Disorders in PACES 83
Case 10: Acromegaly 84
Case 11: Assessment of Thyroid Function, Goitres 88
Case 12: Cushing's Syndrome 93
Dermatology for PACES 97
Case 13: Neurofibromatosis 98
Case 14: Tuberous Sclerosis 101
Vital Tips for Ophthalmology in PACES 103
Case 15: Annual Diabetic Review and Diabetic Retinopathy 104
Case 16: Retinitis Pigmentosa 111

Systemic Examinations (Stations 1B, 3A, 3B & 4B)   113

Station 1B — Respiratory System   115

Introduction to the Respiratory Examination for Paces 115
Case 1: The Surgical Chest 118
    1A — Pneumonectomy & Lobectomy 118
    1B — Old TB & Thoracoplasty 120
    1C — The Lung Transplantation Patient 122
Case 2: Clubbing With Crackles 123
    2A — Bronchiectasis 124
    2B — Pulmonary Fibrosis 126
Case 3: Dullness At The Lung Bases 128
    3A — Pleural Effusion 128
    3B — Consolidation 129
Case 4: Chronic Obstructive Airway Disease 130

Station 3A: Cardiology   133

Introduction to Cardiology 133
Case 1: Prosthetic Heart Valves 135
Case 2: Aortic Stenosis 137
Case 3: Aortic Regurgitation 139
Case 4: Mitral Stenosis 141
Case 5: Pansystolic Murmurs 143
    5A — Mitral Incompetence 143
    5B — Tricuspid Regurgitation 146
    5C — Venricular Septal Defects 148

Station 3B: Neurology — 151

Introduction to the Neurology Section — 151
Neurological Examination of Limbs — 2W2P Method — 152
Examining Speech — The 2W2P Method — 155
Case 1: Extrapyramidal Syndrome — 157
Case 2: Myotonic Dystrophy — 159
Case 3: Cerebellar Syndrome — 161
Case 4: Peripheral Neuropathy — 163
    4A: Charcot Marie Tooth Disease — 166
    4B: Common Peroneal Nerve Palsy — 167
Case 5: Myasthenia Gravis — 168
Case 6: Absent Ankle Jerk With Extensor Planters — 171
    6A — Motor Neuron Disease — 172
    6B — Friedrich's Ataxia — 175
    6C — Subacute Combined Degeneration of the Cord — 176
Case 7: Syringomyelia — 178
Case 8: Spastic Paraparesis — 180
Case 9: Internuclear Ophthalmoplegia — 182
Case 10: Cranial Nerve Syndromes — 186
    10A — Optic Atrophy & Marcus Gunn Pupil — 186
    10B — Oculomotor and Abducens Nerve Lesions — 188
    10C — Facial Palsy — 190
Case 11: Pupillary Abnormalities — 191
    11A — Horner's Syndrome — 191
    11B — Adie's Tonic Pupil — 192
    11C — Argyll Robertson Pupil — 193
Case 12: Hemiplegia — 194

Station 4B: Abdomen — 197

Introduction — 197
Case 1: Patient on Renal Replacement Therapy — 199
Supplementary Case: Autosomal Dominant Polycystic Kidney Disease — 201
Case 2: Patient With Chronic Liver Disease — 203
Additional Case: Haemochromatosis — 207
Additional Case: Liver Transplant — 208
Case 3: Splenomegaly — 209

Index — 213

The contents of this work are intended as a revision aid to the MRCP(UK) PACES examination to aid further understanding and for discussion only. They are not intended and should not be relied upon as recommending a specific clinical method, diagnostic test, or treatment by medical practitioners for any particular patient.

This work has been put together to the best of the authors knowledge and experience, having sat and successfully passed the examination. That said, the publisher and the authors make no representations or warranties with respect to the accuracy or completeness of the contents of this work.

In view of ongoing research, and changes to national treatment guidelines, the reader is urged to review and evaluate up to date information which might supersede the material within this text.

Where relevant, organisations and websites have been cited as a source for further information — this is to provide additional learning resources and evidence, and should not be deemed as an endorsement of the organisation or website quoted. At the time of writing, all internet websites referenced within this book are up to date and relevant, but may be subject to change following publication of this work, altering their content, and hence their applicability to the points made.

PREFACE

The MRCP (UK) examination is continuously changing, reflecting the changing pressures on doctors in training. Whilst the MRCP PACES examination has evolved with the times, the core ethos of it; to act as a benchmark for sound clinical examination, logical diagnostic ability, common sense and most importantly the development of compassionate and ethical physicians has remained unchanged.

Whilst this exam has often struck fear into the hearts of junior doctors, we believe it is an assessment of progression during a physician's training that should be relished as an opportunity to demonstrate these ageless qualities that caring practitioners should possess. This book was born out of the philosophy that all doctors sitting their MRCP PACES already have the knowledge and skill to pass the exam, but just require guidance in the correct logical approach that the Royal College is looking for. The book has therefore, quite unlike other MRCP PACES books, avoided any attempts at being a definitive text. Rather, it has focused on the key aspects that the authors believe are required to pass the examination. Whilst medicine is indeed an ocean, the most commonly examined topics have been selected to reflect the likely scenarios a candidate will face- as the adage goes; "common things occur commonly".

In producing this book, extensive feedback was sought from candidates revising for the examination to reflect their needs. The layout therefore involves a methodical approach with a short introduction, like that presented in the exam, followed by clinical findings expected to be found. Questions likely to be asked and succinct answers have been offered to augment learning. This allows the text to therefore be used both by the bedside with a colleague or in the privacy of one's home to test oneself in the current examination format.

Particular attention has been made to cater for the new PACES 2020/1 format focusing on the novel communication skills stations (Station 1A & 4A) and extended consultations (Station 2 and 5). The new format involves:

- Station 1A: 10 minute communication encounter
- Station 1B: 10 minute respiratory case
- Station 2: 20 minute clinical consultation

- Station 3A: 10 minute cardiology case
- Station 3B: 10 minute neurology case
- Station 4A: 10 minute communication encounter
- Station 4B: 10 minute abdominal case
- Station 5: 20 minute clinical consultation

Station 1A and 4A no longer includes a viva component and will be judged by observation alone.

Station 2 and Station 5 now involve a 15 minutes structured history, examination, explanation of likely diagnosis and management and addressing any questions or concerns followed by a 5 minute viva. The cases for these stations will likely involve diagnoses from the old Station 2 (History taking) and Station 5 (Brief Clinical Consultations) similar to previous iterations of the examination.

We therefore expect these stations to typically involve some kind of multisystem disorder (connective tissue disorders, dermatology, endocrinology themed cases). However, you should expect to be tested on common cases one would encounter during an acute medical take and other cases from Stations 1, 3 & 4.

There remains a focus in the 20 minute clinical consultation on all criteria of the PACES mark scheme focusing on aspects such as maintaining patient welfare and managing concerns. Please familiarise yourself with the mark scheme and details of domains assessed in each station from the MRCP (UK) website. There are seven domains in total and all of them are assessed in Stations 2 & 5 which constitutes over a third of the marks for the whole examination. Therefore, it becomes difficult to pass the exam if one performs poorly in these stations.

In preparation for the examination and writing this textbook, we reviewed every MRCP (PACES) guide available at present and aimed to create a book in the shortest & most palatable format to prepare for the examination in the shortest possible time. The book has been formatted as per the PACES 2020 structure and provides certain special features such as aide memoires in the form of mnemonics and tables written by the authors following years of study. It also contains tips relevant to topics where candidates struggle in exams, especially regarding situations which are common in MRCP (UK) and useful for practical purposes but not adequately covered in any other textbooks. Therefore, we would request you to read the introduction to every section.

Of note is the use of sample presentations and management plans to be memorized by the candidate and adjusted according to the findings of the patient in front of them. Examiners are experienced at recognizing the well prepared from the unprepared candidate. A 'slick' examination followed by a 'slick' & practised presentation often makes the difference between a borderline versus a clear pass. Doing well in the common stations discussed in this book can enable you to pass the exam even if you do poorly in one or two stations.

Never forget to be yourself in the exam — it will both relax you as well as endear you to your examiners and patients alike. It must be remembered that there is no substitute for bedside practice. On the day of the examination, it is imperative that examinees develop the ability to forget about what happened at a station and move on.

Medicine is an art that requires practice. We wish you all the best with your exam and hope that the layout of this book will act to compliment this practice, polishing your approach to the exam.

"Excellence is an art won by training and habituation. We do not act rightly because we have virtue or excellence, but we rather have those because we have acted rightly. We are what we repeatedly do. Excellence, then, is not an act but a habit" — Aristotle.

ABOUT THE AUTHORS

Dr. Hasan Haboubi graduated from Imperial College London in 2006 and completed his early training in the North West Thames Deanery. He was an academic gastroenterology trainee in the Wales Deanery and currently works as a consultant gastroenterologist at University Hospital Llandough, Cardiff and Clinical Lecturer in Swansea University School of Medicine. He has been heavily involved in teaching at both undergraduate and postgraduate levels.

Dr. Nafees Ali graduated from the University of Dhaka, Bangladesh in 2008 and completed his Core Medical Training in the Wales Deanery. He is a Commonwealth Scholar and has developed a passion for medical education. He has been heavily involved in teaching on and organising MRCP (UK) courses. He also teaches on multiple undergraduate programmes.

Dr. Aseel Al-Ansari graduated from Cambridge University with a degree in Medical Sciences and went on to complete clinical studies at Imperial College London in 2008. She is currently a Specialist Registrar in Neurology in the Wales Deanery.

ACKNOWLEDGEMENT

The authors are grateful to Dr James Cronin, Associate Professor, Swansea University for production of the retinal images for this book.

COMMUNICATION ENCOUNTERS
(STATIONS 1A & 4A)

Introduction

This is one of the stations in which people perform poorly in the PACES exam, but it need not be.

There are some essential aspects which the candidate should be aware of, but otherwise most of the cases one will be presented will require the candidate to demonstrate a common-sense approach in order to maintain the patient's best interests.

Here we will highlight some essential aspects of ethical and legal frameworks for the candidate and then illustrate these points through some cases.

Ethics

Principles of Hippocratic ethics

When balancing a difficult ethical decision, it is worth considering four main domains:

Autonomy:
- Principle of self-determination
- Recognition of patients' rights

Non-maleficence:
- Deliberate avoidance of harm

Beneficence:
- Provides the patient with some benefit

Justice:
- The fair and equitable provision of available medical resources to all

You will do well in your discussion with the patient to demonstrate consideration of these 4 domains to the listening examiner.
For example:

1. Autonomy — Demonstrate respect towards patient's wishes and agree shared management plans.

2. Non maleficence — Make clear any suggested any suggested management plans are undertaken in a manner which reduces harmful impact to the patient and/or society.
3. Beneficence — Considering benefits and risks in an empathetic manner.
4. Justice — Try to verbally demonstrate a holistic consideration of all management options and how they might be balanced practically.

Capacity

Assessment of capacity must consider:

- Ability to understand information
- Ability to retain information relating to the decision to be made
- Ability to use or weigh that information as part of the process of making the decision
- Ability to communicate that decision

A doctor who overrides a refusal of treatment is liable to battery (unlawful physical contact) — even if the non-treatment results in death.

A case which illustrates this is Ms B (2002)

- *This was a case of a paralysed ventilator dependent patient who asked doctors to withdraw treatment. They refused but the court judged that she was competent and that the doctors were acting unlawfully in maintaining ventilation.*
- Right to refuse medical intervention is absolute
- No right to consent/demand certain interventions

A case to remember here is that of Dr Nigel Cox (1992)

- Administered Potassium chloride to a patient who had repeatedly requested that he end her life
    - Convicted of attempted murder
- A patient has no right to assisted suicide in the United Kingdom
    - Diane Pretty (2002)
    - Tony Nicholson — lost right to die case in high court

In summary the right to live is not equal to the right to die

Incompetence/lack of capacity

Things to consider:

- Has an advance directive been produced when competent?
- Legally binding if
   - Clearly established
   - Applicable to the circumstances

A doctor who overrides an advance directive is liable to battery

If no advance directive

- Legal duty of the doctor is to act in the patients "best interests"

"Best interests" lacks legal definition.
It is widely accepted that treatment is not in the patient's best interests if it is:

- Futile
- No reasonable hope of therapeutic benefit
- Inflicts excessive burdens on the patient

We will illustrate the ethical dilemmas behind acting in a patient's best interests through the historical case of Tony Bland (1993)

In short, Tony Bland was left in a persistent vegetative state following the 1989 Hillsborough disaster and was fed with an NG tube.

His parents and doctors wanted to withdraw feeding and the hospital applied for judicial declaration that withdrawal would be harmful.

A barrister representing Tony Bland opposed withdrawal of feeding and argued that removing feeding would be murder.

Although the high court and court of appeal initially concluded that withdrawal of feeding would be unlawful, the Law Lords dismissed the court of appeal judgement.
So why was this not murder?

- *Murder is an intentional termination of life by an **act***
- *Withdrawal of feeding tube was an omission.*
- *It was an omission of medical treatment (but not basic care)*
- *There was no obligation to continue treatment because it was not in TB's interests*
- *It was not in his best interests because it was futile.*
- *It was futile because life in a persistent vegetative state was not a benefit in the opinion of a reasonable body of doctors.*

Therefore, the Law lords held that withdrawal of tube feeding was lawful even though they thought that the doctor's intention was to end Mr Bland's life.

Witholding/Withdrawing Life Proloning Treatment

Competent adults

— Patients have the right to refuse treatment even if this results in harm to themselves or death
— Doctors are legally bound to respect their decision
— Patients can express wishes about future treatment in an advance statement

Incompetent adults

— Advance directives are legally binding

IF:

- Made when competent
- Based on adequate information
- Clearly applicable to the present circumstances

It is the doctor's responsibility to decide what is in the patient's best interests when their views are not known

- Seek views of those close to the patient

Difference in view about best interests:

- No legal or ethical obligation to provide treatment if the doctor does not consider it to be clinically indicated
  - Even if a patient specifically requests that treatment
  - Patients have a right to a second opinion
  - This has been challenged in the courts

Difference of view about best interests (incompetent adults)

- Consider the views of doctors, health care team and those close to the patient
- Try to reach a consensus
- Seek a second opinion or independent review
- Seek legal advice if significant difference cannot be resolved
- Can try time limited trials of treatment if clinical uncertainty

The Mental Capacity Act (2005)

There are 5 principles:

1. Assume a person has capacity unless proved otherwise
2. Do not treat people as incapable of making a decision unless all practical steps have been tried to help them
3. A person should not be treated as incapable of making a decision because you deem their decision to be unwise
4. Always do things or take decisions for people without capacity in their best interests
5. Before doing something to someone or making a decision on their behalf, consider whether the outcome could be achieved in a less restrictive way

Capacity Assessment

A capacity assessment must consider:

- Ability to understand information
- Ability to retain information relating to the decision to be made
- Ability to use or weigh that information as part of the process of making the decision
- Ability to communicate above decision

Best Interests

The Act does not define best interests but does give a checklist. The decision maker must:

- involve the person who lacks capacity
- have regard for past and present wishes and feelings, especially written statements
- consult with others who are involved in the care of the person
- not make assumptions based solely on the person's age, appearance, condition or behaviour

Medical treatment requiring court approval

- Withdrawal or withholding of artificial nutrition / fluids in patients with PVS
- Organ or bone marrow donation by a person lacking capacity to consent
- Sterilisation of a person lacking capacity to consent
- Other cases where there is doubt or dispute about whether a treatment will be in a person's best interest

The Independent Mental Capacity Advocate (IMCA)

IMCA's are an extra safeguard for particularly vulnerable people in specific situations

- There is a duty on local authorities or NHS bodies to provide this service where necessary
- IMCA's will be given to people who have no friends or family with whom it is practicable to consult

Communication

There are several important aspects within communication that need to be considered.

You will be assessed on your ability to empathise with your patient so remember, whatever the situation, your patient is the priority of care.

Some simple approaches are mentioned below regarding common situations seen in the exam.

We will provide some worked examples. It is a good idea to practise the scenarios with another colleague before reading through the best practice we have recommended and then making relevant adjustments accordingly. It might be a good idea for you to spend some time with senior colleagues and the palliative care team/nurses and watch them break difficult news and deal with complaints.

Case 1: Breaking Bad News

We suggest you use the SPIKES 6-point approach:

- Setting — Ensuring the patient or relative is at ease and has had the opportunity to include family members in the consultation should they wish. Also ensure the location for the conversation is appropriate and that you are well versed with the case. Do your best to maximise on verbal (empathetic tone) and non-verbal communication skills (good eye contact, etc.)
- Perception — Start off by clarifying what the patient or relative already knows. This allows you also to gauge a patient's perception regarding the illness.
- Invitation — Establish what the patient wants to know and in how much detail. Examples of statements used include: "Would you like me to go into some detail about what we think has happened/is going on?"
- Knowledge — Deliver the patient the knowledge regarding the bad news. This is best done by giving a warning shot first such as "I'm sorry that I have some bad news for you". You can then break the bad news gently, e.g. talking about abnormalities and then explaining what they are.
- Empathy — Leave a short period of silence after delivering the bad news, then acknowledge the patient's natural feeling of being upset. Try to evaluate what it is about the diagnosis that is making them feel distressed (effect on family, fear of condition, etc), then try to offer support for these specific feelings.
- Strategy and Summary: Summarise how things can be taken forward, and the support mechanisms that will be available along the way.

For other situations such as admitting fault and possible harm to a patient, you can still follow this approach, focussing on identifying what is known first, clarifying in an empathetic or apologetic way and then summarising an action plan to take things forward and ensure such events don't happen again. We will illustrate some scenarios in the subsequent cases.

A worked example follows.

Instructions to examinee: *You review a 35-year-old lady who was recently under your care with an atypical pneumonia. As part of her work up she has HIV testing which has returned positive. She is a married mother of two. You bring her back to clinic to discuss the results.*

There are many aspects that need to be explored in such as case and SPIKES is a useful tool for this.

- Setting — Ensure the setting is correct to have this discussion. Ask if she wishes to have anyone here.
- Perception — Review the patients understanding of why the test was performed and in what context.
- Invitation — Establish that the patient wishes to know the results. A statement like "As you may recall we were performing a number of tests to identify why you had a pneumonia and some of them were to look for conditions such as HIV which would make you more at risk of chest infections. I have some of the results here today which I can go through with you if that's what you would like"
- Knowledge — Empathetically inform the patient regarding the positive result. Use verbal and non-verbal cues to comfort the patient.
- Empathy — Allow the patient the space to vent their emotions. There will be a mix of anger, frustration, shock and denial. The key thing is to listen. You are not going to be able to alleviate all these feelings, nor should you try to. Your job is to be supportive and help the patient to focus on the next aspects of care.
- Strategy & Summary — You will need to come up with a management plan for the patient — this will involve referral to the infectious diseases team to start HAART. Remember there is a taboo associated with a diagnosis of HIV, but patient's life expectancies are not significantly altered by the diagnosis so long as they are compliant with their medication and follow-up. The difficulty of this case may also come in the follow-up of other family members. You may wish to evaluate this with a question such as "Do you know how you may have acquired the infection" and "Do you have any reason to suspect that any other individuals may have acquired the infection too"

In this case there are also issues which may arise such as how the patient contracted HIV and testing of family members.

There is now another issue of confidentiality which needs to be reviewed here.

The following list includes situations when confidentiality can be broken:

- Legal duty — When requested by a court order
- Statutory duty — Informing of communicable diseases, births, deaths, etc.
- Public duty —
    - National security reasons such as terrorism or major crime
    - When a third party may be at risk (i.e. someone at risk of communicable disease)
    - Where public may be at risk (e.g. informing the DVLA about the risks of a patient driving)

Where possible, you should encourage patients to have discussions with relatives regarding the diagnosis. Whilst loss of trust and breakdown of the doctor patient relationship can occur if you breach confidentiality without the patient's consent, you have a responsibility to do so in situations where others are at risk.

In such difficult situations, you can offer a compromise such as bringing in the spouse to discuss the diagnosis together.

Case 2: The Angry Relative/Complaints

Here we demonstrate how the above approach can be modified to speak to an angry relative.

A worked example follows.

You speak to the relatives of a patient who received Amiodarone for an "abnormal heart rhythm" many years ago following a myocardial infarction. The patient now has pulmonary fibrosis.

Suggest using the SPIKES approach:

- **Setting** — Ensuring the patient or relative is at ease and has had the opportunity to include family members in the consultation should they wish.
- **Perception** — Clarify what is already known about the management following the heart attack and what has been explained thus far regarding the patient's lung condition.
- **Invitation** — Establish what the relative wants to know and in how much detail.
- **Knowledge** — Deliver the patient the knowledge regarding the bad news. This is best done by giving a warning shot first such as "I'm sorry that I have some bad news for you". You can then break the bad news gently, e.g. talking about abnormalities and then explaining what they are.
- **Empathy** — Leave a short period of silence after delivering the bad news, then acknowledge the patients natural feeling of being upset. Try to evaluate what it is about the diagnosis that is making them feel distressed (effect on family, fear of condition, etc), then try to offer support for these specific feelings.
- **Strategy and Summary:** Summarise how things can be taken forward

There are some key concepts in communicating with angry patients or relatives that are important to be aware of:

1. You must acknowledge concerns, even if you feel they are unreasonable.
2. You must try to deal with the emotions of the patient or relative before turning your attention to the facts of the case (remember this is a communication station so the examiners are not as interested in your knowledge of the management but more in how you deal with the patient's or relative's concerns).

3. Do not criticise colleagues or previous management plans — you were not present and therefore are unable to comment on the details. If an angry patient or relative tries to push you in to incriminating colleagues, you are better off avoiding this discussion with a statement such as "As I wasn't present during the decision-making process regarding your treatment, I can't comment on the thoughts of the attending doctors at that point in time. I would prefer to focus our consultation today on aspects that we can directly affect today and how we can take your management forward".
4. If you do not know a management plan, it is best to be honest about this and tell the patient or relative that you will make it your priority to find out immediately after the consultation has ended and relay that information to them. Perhaps also consider offering to take their telephone number to call them back.
5. Patients and relatives are entitled to make formal complaints if they so wish and your job is not to persuade them not to. Your job in this station is to investigate their ideas, concerns and expectations and empathetically deal with them.

If they ask for your assistance in making a formal complaint, you should direct them to the Patients Advice and Liaison Services (PALS) who will be able to take the complaint forward.

Case 3: Fitness To Drive

Example Case:
You see a 52-year-old man who has recently been admitted with tonic-clonic seizures.

He is reviewed by the neurology team and the history and EEG's are felt to be suggestive of idiopathic generalised epilepsy. You are asked to discuss this diagnosis with him.

Here you will find the patient is a lorry driver and will be at risk of loss of earnings because of restrictions to his driving.

There are several aspects you need to be aware of in such a case.

Driving Restrictions

Enclosed are a summary of DVLA driving restrictions:
Car driver:
If you have had epileptic attacks whilst being awake and lost consciousness:

- You will not be allowed to drive.
- You can reapply for a licence if you have been seizure free for 1-year.
- If seizures triggered by change in anti-epileptic medication (changed drug or lowered dose), you can reapply if seizure free for 6-months.
- A one-off seizure while awake within which you have lost consciousness: Not allowed to drive unless seizure free for 6-months, or 12-months if a cause found that may increase risk.

Seizures whilst asleep: The DVLA may let you keep your licence if the attacks are only when the patient is asleep and the time from the first attack is more than 12-months (i.e. less likely to now have daytime attacks).

Seizures that do not affect consciousness: The DVLA may let the patient keep their licence if these are the only attacks and the time from the first attack is more than 12-months.

HGV Driver:
More than one seizure: Not allowed to drive unless seizure free for 10-years and/or been off anti-epileptics for 10-years.

One off seizure: Not allowed to drive unless seizure free for 5-years and have not taken any anti-epileptics for 5-years.

Confidentiality

You will need to review the patient's intentions to inform the DVLA.

If the patient refuses to inform the DVLA, you will need to let the patient know that you will be legally and morally obliged to do so.

Communication

Using the SPIKES approach, this consultation needs to be delivered empathetically.

In "Perception" you should investigate how this makes the patient feel, and what impact it will have on their work and family.

In "Strategy" you can think of this as short term: how is the patient going to get home from the clinic, to medium term: offer to write a medical letter to the patient's employer supporting their change of role to one that does not involve driving or operating machinery, e.g. an office job.

Longer term strategies will obviously be dictated by the patient's ability to drive and you should offer to meet the patient again to review and discuss this. Lengths of restrictions are detailed below.

The following conditions are notifiable to the DVLA:

- Epilepsy
- Strokes
- Physical disabilities that may limit driving
- Neurological conditions that may limit driving
- Visual impairments

Notification does not mean not being allowed to drive. It requires individual assessment by the DVLA

Specific situations: For full details, please consult the up-to-date DVLA guidelines: https://www.gov.uk/driving-medical-conditions

TIA/Stroke

- Car: Stop driving for 1-month
- HGV: Stop driving for 1-year
- If still symptomatic following a stroke you must tell the DVLA

Ischaemic Heart Disease

Group 1 licence (car) holders with angina do not need to involve the DVLA unless symptomatic behind the wheel, but Group 2 licence holders (HGV) must.

Car:
- Stop driving for 1-week if you have had angioplasty/stents and it was successful and no further treatment is required
- Stop driving for 4-weeks if you have had angioplasty/stents but unsuccessful and further treatment required
- Stop driving for 4-weeks if MI (STEMI or NSTEMI) which was not treated with angioplasty

HGV Driver:
- Stop driving for 6-weeks
- Medical assessment after 6-weeks to review fitness to drive

CABG:
- Car: Stop driving for 4-weeks
- HGV: Stop driving for 3-months

IDDM

All insulin dependent diabetics must inform the DVLA if their insulin treatment will last more than 3 months. All patients should check their blood sugar before driving and every 2-hours whilst driving.

Car:
- No restrictions if aware of symptoms of hypoglycaemia and no significant retinopathy/visual impairment.
- Licence may be revoked if >1 incidence of hypoglycaemia in the preceding 12 months requiring the assistance of others.

HGV: Restricted — not allowed to drive, but can apply for licence, pending the following:
- No episodes of hypoglycaemia at the wheel within the last 12 months
- Receive an assessment from a diabetes consultant at least once a year
- Regularly test your blood glucose levels, especially before and around times of driving
- Have stable blood sugar control on insulin for at least a month
- Have no other conditions that would invalidate an application for the license
- Sign a declaration to follow doctor's decisions and report any significant changes in your condition to the DVLA

Case 4: Industrial Injury Benefits

You review a 72-year old — man who was recently an inpatient on your ward with a unilateral effusion. You are asked to see him in clinic with the results.

His CT scan shows pleural thickening and plaques and pleural aspirate cytology shows large clusters of cells displaying a mesothelial phenotype with a low nuclear: cytoplasmic ratio and knobbly edges consistent with malignant mesothelioma. There is also evidence of peritoneal deposits.

Approach:

This is essentially a breaking bad news consultation, although there is a twist which candidates need to be aware of and explore, namely that of an occupational injury.

The breaking bad news SPIKES approach will work well for this case (and all such cases where the patient is receiving a result or information that has the potential to shock/upset them).

- Setting — After introducing yourself to the patient and clarifying the purpose of the consultation (namely to review them with the results of their recent investigations), enquire if they wish to have anyone else with them to help understand the results.
- Perception — Review the patients understanding of why the test was performed and in what context. You should recap the history of their admission with breathlessness which culminated with the diagnosis of "fluid on the lung" which you have been trying to identify a cause for.
- Invitation — Establish that the patient wishes to know the results.
- Knowledge — Empathetically inform the patient regarding the positive result. Use verbal and non-verbal cues to comfort the patient. Explain that the diagnosis is that of a lung cancer which you believe to be related to previous asbestos exposure. You may need to explore the occupational history in brief — nature and duration of exposure but do not labour these points as it is not the purpose of this consultation.
- Empathy — Allow the patient the space to express their feelings. There will be emotions of shock and worry. Remember to give the patient time here. Do not be afraid to allow a period of silence as well. Make good eye contact, lean forward and nod your head slowly in an empathetic manner.

- Strategy & Summary — Following the breaking of bad news, you will need to explain the implications of the results. The patient's case will be discussed at a lung multidisciplinary team (MDT) meeting. This includes respiratory physicians, thoracic surgeons, oncologists, radiologists, pathologists and specialist nurses. The patient may ask you about prognosis. It is difficult to comment without discussion at an MDT, but if appropriate you can explain that there is no known cure for this but that treatments including chemotherapy, radiotherapy and biological therapies can improve survival outcomes. The patient will be contacted by a member of the MDT to discuss management plans following the meeting.

You will also need to discuss compensation with the patient which is something specific to this case. Check if the patient is aware first and explain that they may be eligible to claim for industrial disablement benefit. The process for this is for the patient to obtain a form B1 from their local social services. This form covers occupational lung diseases. Following this, a medical officer may visit to assess degree of disability. Given that there has also been a discussion of breaking bad news in this consultation, it would be worth offering to write this information down for the patient. Before closing the consultation, remember to recap the consultation and the agreed strategy forward. Don't forget to invite any other concerns.

The following lung conditions are eligible for compensation:

- Coal workers pneumoconiosis
- Silicosis
- Mesothelioma
- Asbestosis
- Bilateral diffuse pleural thickening
- Primary lung cancer with evidence of asbestosis

*Isolated asbestos related pleural plaques are not covered within the industrial disablement benefit.

Case 5: Negligence

You meet with a 52-year old man who suffered a myocardial infarction 13-years ago. His stay in hospital at that time was complicated by episodes of ventricular arrhythmias and he was started on Amiodarone with good effect. He has been complaining of breathlessness for some months and recent investigations have shown he has pulmonary fibrosis, presumed to be related to his Amiodarone. You meet him in the Cardiology outpatient clinic to inform him of these findings. The patient claims that he was not told about potential complications.

Approach:

The approach to all communication stations is to clarify the understanding of the patient/relative you are meeting, then deliver the information required, then review and recap. This case is an example of an adverse event which will result in a complaint.

You can use an abbreviated form of the SPIKES consultation to deal with this.

- Setting — Acknowledge that the patient is naturally worried about the results of the investigations but clarify that they are willing to have a discussion with you.
- Perception — Clarify what information they already know about what has happened, both in their past medical history and more recently. You will then need to summarise the events that led up to this clinic consultation.
- Knowledge — Explain the results of the investigations and explain that this may be related to the medication that was previously started.
- Empathy — The patient may be angry that they have suffered a life changing side effect as a result of a treatment. The key is to listen without interruption and let the patient express their anger. Remain calm, and take the time to explore their feelings, including fears about how this diagnosis may affect them.

    The patient may wish to issue blame against certain doctors. This may be acceptable, and your job is not to defend actions of individuals but your role in this consultation is to break the bad news and to apologise that potential side effects may not have been explained to the patient. You should acknowledge their anger "I understand that you are upset." You should only deal with facts and if the patient discussed conversations that you have not been part of, you should

listen empathetically but remain neutral and not attribute blame as you were not there.
- Strategy & Summary — You should help the patient have a plan to take things forward. Give assurances that further action will be taken. You will refer them to the respiratory team. You will organise to meet the patient again with their family if necessary, to go through the diagnosis. You should offer to direct them towards the local hospital PALS (Patient Advice and Liaison Service) where they can raise this as a formal complaint. Ensure that you ask about any additional questions or concerns at the end.

Discussion: This case deals with managing a complaint/upset patient.

Key communication skills here are to respect the patient's anger and not try to influence their decision making but support them with their emotions and offer avenues for escalation — this could involve escalating to inform your consultant or registering events as a "clinical incident" or through formal complaints procedures through the patient advice and liaison service.

Knowledge to recap:
There are two levels of complaint:

- Local: these are often resolved within the institution by PALS/local staff and managers.
- NHS Ombudsman: Usually investigate larger incidents or severe administrative failures.

Negligence is a slightly different concept which describes poor clinical practice which results in a negative outcome for a patient.

In short, there are 3 conditions which need to be met for negligence to be attributed.

1. The clinician had a duty of care to the patient.
2. The clinician in question gave suboptimal care. This will be viewed by means of the Bolam test (what would a reasonable body of practitioners do in similar circumstances).
3. This breach of appropriate care resulted in harm to the patient.

There is a time limit for raising questions of negligence which is set at within 3 years of the act of alleged negligence.

Case 6: Discussing Organ Donation

You are working in the Intensive Care Unit looking after a 35-year old lady who was admitted the night before with headache and collapse. A CT scan showed a large subarachnoid haemorrhage with mass effect and evidence of herniation. The patient is intubated and ventilated but neurological assessment shows absence of brain stem function. You are asked to speak to the husband about stopping ventilatory support and considering organ donation as a donor card was found in her purse.

Approach:

There are two parts to this consultation. The first part of this communication station requires breaking bad news. The spouse knows the diagnosis, but you should still use the SPIKES approach to clarify what is known and emphasise that this is an un-survivable intracranial event.

Make sure you have tackled all aspects of this before moving on to any discussion on organ donation. In short:

- Setting — Ensure that the husband has all the support he needs.
- Perception & Invitation — Clarify his understanding of the what has happened and willingness to know outcomes of assessments.
- Knowledge– Inform him that you have conducted assessments of brain stem function and discussed the case with the neurosurgical team who have suggested that this injury is fatal. You will need to clarify that this means that the patient is dead and that her organs are only working because of the support her body is getting from the ventilator.
- Empathy — Ensure you pause and use all verbal and non-verbal cues to ensure bad news is delivered in the most empathetic way.
- Strategy & Summary — You will need to utilise this segment of the consultation to move into discussions on organ donation.

One example of a statement would be "I appreciate this is an awful time for you. I'm so very sorry. But there is something else that we wanted to discuss with you if that is ok? Were you aware that your wife carried an organ donation card?" From such a statement you can engage in a conversation about what organ donation is and what the next steps may be. They will need to know that:

- The patient will have additional blood tests, including for viruses such as Hepatitis and HIV to identify any potential infections which could affect organ function.

- An operation will need to be undertaken to obtain the organs for transplant
- Not all organs may be used. This is dependent on other factors, including on the recipient's side of the transplant.

In your summary, you should give them some information and offer to put them in touch with the transplant coordinator. Be aware that this is an emotionally challenging time and whilst decisions regarding organ donation do need to be made in a timely manner, the husband should be offered time to think about things.

Knowledge to recap:

The Human Tissue Act (1961) and Human Organ Transplant Act (1989) govern the code of practice for organ retrieval and transplant. They also comment on establishment of brain stem death, namely:

1) The patient must have had all reversible causes excluded
2) There is no spontaneous respiratory drive
3) There must be no response to brainstem reflexes such as the pupil, corneal, vestibulo-ocular, gag and cough reflexes.

Organs are preferably retrieved as "beating-heart" as this optimises the chances of successful transplant. Aside from known HIV or prior disease, other contraindications include variant CJD and disseminated malignancy.

Case 7: Gillick Competence

You are asked to meet the mother of a patient who is under your care. She is a 16-year old girl who was been having painful periods and has been using non-steroidal anti-inflammatory drugs to assist with this. She was admitted with an upper gastrointestinal bleed and requires a blood transfusion prior to endoscopy. Her mother is a Jehovah's witness and does not want her daughter to receive a transfusion but the patient is happy to receive a transfusion.

Approach: You should start this case by ensuring you show your awareness of the mother's concern given the stressful situation. An example statement may be "I appreciate you are very worried about the bleeding that your daughter has had and have asked to speak to me about some of the treatments that we are planning on offering."

You should also clarify that consent has been given by the daughter to speak to the mother about her care, as she is over 16-years old and has capacity to make decisions so should be treated as such. You should listen caringly as the mother explains her wish for her daughter to not receive a transfusion in favour of other resuscitative products. It is important not to interrupt and to give the parent the time she needs to discuss her ideas, concerns and expectations.

Following this you should calmly state that you must respect the patient's wishes and that she would like to have a blood transfusion. You should again pause and allow for this information to distil and be open and confident enough to any invite questions regarding this.

Knowledge to Recap:
There are three main issues that will be assessed in such a scenario.

1. Knowledge of consent for the patient to allow you to speak to relatives
2. Knowledge that patient is Gillick Competent and can consent to treatment without their parent's approval.
3. Good communication skills. The mother may become upset or even angry at your rejection of her request to give intravenous crystalloid instead of blood. You will need to show empathy towards her beliefs, but also show that the patient is your priority and that you are legally and morally obliged to do what is in her best interests and in accordance with her wishes.

Case 8: Life Insurance And Genetic Disorders

A 22-year old lady is seen in the outpatient clinic. Her mother and three of her sisters have been diagnosed with breast cancer. You are asked to speak to her about her recent genetic testing results. You will need to report to her that she is BRCA1 gene positive and discuss the implications of this with her.

Progress: During the consultation she mentions she has life insurance but that she doesn't want to inform her insurance company.
Approach:
There are 3 key aspects to this consultation.

1. You will need to employ a breaking bad news strategy and could use the SPIKES approach in order to facilitate this.
2. You will need to employ the principles of genetic counselling here.
   - These require that a good history and pedigree construction is made
   - Clinical examination is undertaken
   - Genetic tests are appropriately performed
   - Counselling is performed for positive results — the aim is not to reduce the incidence of a genetic disease in the future but to help the individual and their family cope with the diagnosis
   - Simple structured information sheets should be offered at the end.
   - There are implications to this diagnosis in terms of risk of developing breast cancer which will need to be explored. There is a 72% lifetime risk of developing breast cancer in BRCA1 positive women and 69% risk in BRCA2 positive women. You will therefore need to discuss options that the patient may consider — this could include surveillance but would also include the prospect of a prophylactic mastectomy. Given the implications of this in a young woman about to go travelling, this will need to be visited in a sensitive manner.
3. The patient doesn't want to inform the insurance company. Important aspects here are that you don't have any authority to break confidentiality here and if the patient doesn't wish to inform the insurance company, they can choose to do so. The situations where confidentiality can be broken relate to patients at risk to other individuals or the community, for example in the case of

serious transmittable illnesses, but this is not the case here. You may be asked about whether the insurance company has the right to access her medical records.

The Association of British Insurances (ABI) genetic testing code of conduct states the following:

- No insurer can request an applicant undertake a genetic test
- When applying for life insurance, individuals can apply for up to £500,000 without informing the insurance company. When applying for critical illness insurance, individuals can apply for up to £300,000 without informing the insurance company
- However, if the individual applies for insurance of greater than £500,000, their genetic diagnosis will not be used in the assessment of their application unless it is specifically in the applicant's favour.

An important genetic illness to be aware of and commonly tested in the examination is:

- Huntington's disease — Autosomal dominant inheritance, associated with a CAG trinucleotide repeat which results in a mutated form of the Huntington protein. This results in chorea, cognitive impairment and psychiatric symptoms.

CLINICAL CONSULTATIONS (STATIONS 2 & 5)

Introduction

The clinical consultations stations 2 & 5 gives the candidate the opportunity to demonstrate the full range of clinical competences, namely history taking, focused clinical examination, generation of appropriate differential diagnoses, knowledge of management strategies, communication and shared decision making in an empathetic manner. These stations constitute over a third of the marks for the whole exam with assessment of all seven clinical skills.

It can be a lot easier than you anticipate because these stations represent most closely what you do in real life. The format of this station is new to the PACES 2020 examination. In each station you will have 15 minutes to conduct your clinical consultation with the patient followed by a five-minute viva. You should ideally spend 5–7 minutes on the history, 4–5 minutes on the focused clinical examination and 4–5 minutes on discussing with the patients any ideas, concerns and expectations they have, management plans, safety netting and follow up.

In this chapter, we will review history taking in general first and then comment on any specific medical history questions under the relevant case. In the second half of this chapter we will discuss some cases that formed the short cases section in the old PACES examination and were often examined in the brief clinical consultations station as these are favourite cases amongst examiners and likely to return in this new format.

History taking is the basis of clinical medicine. However, when you are preparing for PACES, it is very important to have a clear structure in this process so that you can obtain a full history, create a problem list, give the patient a plan and address their concerns within a 15-minute window. At 12-minutes into the consultation, you may be given a warning. At this point, *it is imperative that you start **summarising to the patient** what you think is going on and **explain your plan** including any investigations you want to do briefly and then make **follow up plans** with results and after discussion with seniors/specialists.* A well-rounded knowledge of clinical medicine is essential and hopefully you will have acquired the requisite skills for this station during preparation for Part 1 and Part 2 written and by working in a busy Medical Assessment Unit. Expect cases from other stations to be modified into clinical consultations.

The key lies in **using the 5 minutes before you go into the stations to prepare.** Read through the scenarios quickly and make a list of differential diagnoses for the problem in question using a standard "surgical sieve". Planning individual cases, practising with colleagues, attending clinics, and working on a busy medical assessment unit is the way to prepare for these stations. When practising or seeing patients on your on-calls and clinics, set a timer on your mobile phone and check if you are able to complete your consultation within 15 minutes.

Take a full history using the following mnemonic:

3PMAFTOSA —

- Presenting Complaints
- Past Medical & Surgical History
- Personal History
- Medications
- Allergies
- Family history
- Travel
- Occupation
- Social History
- A review of systems and 'Anything else I may have overlooked'?

Always start with an open question. During that first minute, try to listen without interrupting.

When you go into the details Presenting Complaints, or history of present illness, for pain, use the mnemonic **SOCRATES** (Site, Onset, Character, Radiation, Associated features, Timing, Exacerbating & Relieving Factors, Severity).

For every other symptom, use **ODPARA** (Onset, Duration, Progression, Aggravating factors, Relieving factors, Associated Features).

The associated features should include relevant symptoms to that system.

- Cardiovascular system: Chest Pain, Dyspnoea, Syncope/Presyncope, Palpitations (get patients to tap out the rhythm), Orthopnoea, PND, Ankle swelling, Fatigue, Family history of sudden cardiac deaths (if another relevant cardiac symptom).

- Respiratory system: **CWSH** — Cough, Chest pain (especially pleuritic), Wheeze, Weight loss, Stridor, Sputum, SOB, Haemoptysis.
- Gastrointestinal system:
  Upper GI — Dysphagia, Odynophagia, Reflux/Dyspepsia, Haematemesis/Melaena, Vomiting.

  Lower GI — Changes in bowel habits, Abdominal pain, PR bleeding.

  Liver — Jaundice, Change in colour of urine and stool, Pruritus.

  Constitutional symptoms — Weight loss, Fatigue and Lethargy (symptoms of anaemia), Appetite
- Genitourinary: Haematuria; Dysuria; Lower urinary tract symptoms (Urgency; Hesitancy; Terminal dribbling; Poor stream; Feeling of incomplete evacuation; Painful or slow stream; Incontinence; Nocturia); Loin pain; Genital discharge; Sexual problems. Please do not forget to take a history of abnormal uterine bleeding in women.
- Neurology: SOCRATES for headaches. ODPARA for Muscular weakness; Paraesthesia; Visual Disturbance; Speech Disturbance (see Station 3); Dysphagia; Involuntary movements & Tremors; Seizures/Fits; Syncope and Vertigo/Dizziness; AMTS; Sphincter disturbance.

After obtaining a relevant history, do a focussed examination pertinent to the problem in question. Sometimes, it can be challenging. Especially in cases involving multisystem disease, for example vasculitides, examiners will penalise you if there is a symptom such as sensorineural hearing loss or loss of vision and you have not had time to examine it.

With most station 2 & 5 cases (and some neurology cases in Station 3 e.g. Parkinson's disease; Cerebellar dysfunction), you need to **PLAN THE COMMON CASES IN ADVANCE AND PRACTISE WITH YOUR COLLEAGUES THE SPECIFIC ORDER IN WHICH YOU ARE GOING ASK QUSTIONS AND EXAMINE** thereby demonstrating your understanding of what is relevant to that case. We shall provide a method for most of the subsections for you to use but feel free to improvise as this is not a rigid structure.

In the latter part of this chapter we will describe in greater detail how to take a history of musculoskeletal/rheumatology problems, endocrinopathies and relevant dermatology cases for the exam.

Check how things are at home & work. Has the disease affected the patient's livelihood or independence with activities of daily living? Always do your **SYSTEMS REVIEW** (BOWELS, WATERWORKS, SKIN, JOINTS, WEIGHT LOSS, APETITE, SLEEP, MOBILITY). Important clues are hidden in the full history and with practice the last 2 Ps and MAFTOSA can be covered in about 90 seconds.

Ask the patients about their specific **CONCERNS**. Simply asking this question scores you marks from each examiner. Ask them what their **IDEAS** and **EXPECTATIONS** are about what is going on and what **INVESTIGATIONS** and **TREATMENT** they have had for this so far for their problem. Always offer leaflets for chronic conditions. Advise patients not to read from unofficial/non-evidenced websites on the internet but if they want to, they can use the NHS website.

At the end of your consultation, ask yourself if you know the answers to the following questions.

- What is the Condition?
- What is the Cause?
- What Complications has the patient had as a result of this condition?
- How has this affected the patient's functional Capacity i.e. their lives, work etc.
- What is patient's main Concern? Have I addressed it?

If you know the answers to those **5 Cs**, you can give yourself a pat on your back because you will leave a satisfied patient.

Once you've summarised to the patient, explained your plan and arranged follow up, thank the patient, then turn to the examiner and very briefly explain what you've gathered in your history and what diagnosis/differential diagnoses these features are consistent with. Do not ramble. Use a maximum of 30 seconds.

The examiners would have heard the same story over and over and will be bored and a candidate who does not present in a brief, concise manner and rambles does not appear confident and is more likely to fail. Remember they are looking for future registrars who they can rely on to give them a summary about an unwell patient at three in the morning on the telephone.

The examiners have 5 minutes in total and you must give them the opportunity to ask you some questions so that they can cover every skill they are examining you on. Most examiners will have decided what questions they are going to ask every candidate and if you do not give them the opportunity to ask these questions, they cannot give you marks.

Therefore, it is vital to have memorised a sample management plan *"I would like to manage this patient in a multidisciplinary approach with early involvement of specialist physicians, physiotherapy, occupational therapy and rehabilitation services with focus on patient & family education. Specific management involves... (MENTION EDUCATION, LIFESTYLE CHANGES AS WELL AS MEDICAL AND SURGICAL TREATMENT OPTIONS)".*

We have provided some sample cases for you to practise that often come up in exams. However, please understand that the object of these cases is NOT TO TEACH YOU CLINICAL MEDICINE but rather to TEST YOUR HISTORY TAKING SKILLS. We suggest finding colleagues/fellow examinees to practise with.

One case that stresses candidates and often comes up in PACES is ophthalmoscopy. Do not be alarmed if this comes up in the examination. With a few weeks left for the exam, prepare for the two common cases (diabetic nephropathy and retinitis pigmentosa). *Learn to use an ophthalmoscope with an expert.* We will give you some guidance in the relevant chapter as well. It is a good idea to take your own ophthalmoscope to the exam. The green light on your ophthalmoscope brilliantly shows neovascularisation that would not be visible to the naked eye.

Before we finish, in preparation for these stations, we suggest that you plan to do at least one clinic in each of the following specialties at your hospital if you have not already done so.

- Rheumatology: Often a lot of patients come for biologics therapy or joint injections to the day-case unit. Arrange to go and speak to these patients under timed conditions.
- Medical ophthalmology: Choose a clinic where there is going to be some LASER treatment for diabetic retinopathy. Request the specialist to teach you to use the ophthalmoscope.
- Endocrinology & Diabetes: See how diabetic nurse specialists counsel/educate their patients. Make sure you see a case of Acromegaly and learn how to assess thyroid function clinically. Learn about pathologies including Grave's disease, Multinodular goitre, Thyroiditis incl. drug induced cases, Thyroid malignancies and Hashimoto's thyroiditis. You will have seen Addison's and Cushing's

Disease on the wards. <u>Never forget to ask about pituitary surgery and always examine the nose for scars</u>.
- Dermatology: If you can spare time — see some rashes and skin cancers. It is educational.

We assume that you have attended enough clinics in the other specialties relevant to Stations 1B, 3 and 4B. Going to valve clinics, neurology, gastro/hepatology and respiratory medicine outpatient clinics is as useful as spending some time on specialist cardiothoracic and neurosurgery units at the nearest tertiary care hospital to see good pathology. Always introduce yourself to the nurse in charge of the ward you are on and the patient, explain what you are doing (that you are preparing for an examination) and seek permission before proceeding with your practice.

It is better to go around in groups of two or three so that one of you can act as an examiner and prep the patient before one of the others practises under timed conditions.

The basics of clinical medicine remain unchanged: History & examination → Formulate differential diagnoses/a problem list → Investigate to confirm diagnoses/rule out differentials → Communicate to the patient what the disease is → Offer treatment options to the patient.

This is something you do five days a week and when you are on call regularly as a physician. Try to treat the exam as a clinic and the encounters with examiners as a post take ward round and you will sail through the exam. Another useful tip would be to speak to consultants in your hospital who are PACES examiners and request them to supervise practice sessions. Let the on-call team know you are preparing for PACES as well and ask them to page you if any interesting patients with signs are admitted.

Case 1: Headache

Briefing for examinee: You are an SHO in General Internal Medicine clinic. This 67-year-old female patient has been referred by her GP with early morning headaches. She has a background of hypothyroidism, poorly controlled T2DM and hypertension.

Briefing for patient: You are 67 years of age and have been overweight since you were diagnosed with hypothyroidism 10 years ago. You have had an early morning headache for most days in the week for years. The headache gradually gets better through the day. It is usually all over the head and your vision is never affected. The headache is not associated with trauma, sex, meals and not worse on walking, lying down, bending forward or coughing. You are tired all the time and have no energy. Your GP has tested your thyroid function, and this is well controlled. Your diabetes is very well controlled, and you have never had nocturnal hypoglycaemia to the best of your knowledge. You are very aware of the symptoms of hypoglycaemia. Your live with your husband. However, he sleeps in a separate room now because you keep him up with your snoring.

You have not noticed any changes in your appearance and your hands and feet have not grown. You are so tired you often doze off when you sit down in front of the television. You are forgetful. You are a retired secretary. You don't smoke and are a teetotaller. Your mobility is ok. You are post-menopausal. You must wear a pad at times because you can become incontinent. Your GP is concerned. Currently you are on Aspirin 75 mg OD, Atorvastatin 20 mg ON, Gliclazide 160 mg BD, Metformin 1 g BD, Perindopril 4 mg OD. You have no allergies. There is no recent travel history. You are unsure as to what is causing your headache and your main concern is to ensure that you have not had any brain tumours because your neighbour has recently been diagnosed with this condition.

Key issues: Using SOCRATES to take a history of headache and using the associated features to extrapolate a diagnosis of Obstructive sleep apnoea or Obesity Hypoventilation syndrome. It does make a difference in terms of management because OSA is classically treated with CPAP whilst if a patient develops hypercapnic respiratory failure because of either OSA/OHS, he/she might end up needing BIPAP. It is a skill to be able to individually rule out the common benign chronic causes of headache (migraine, cluster, tension headache) as well as headaches related to raised intracranial pressure and rule out red flag symptoms. It is important to think about headaches associated with raised intracranial pressure (headaches worse on lying, bending forward or coughing). Do not forget sinusitis and postnasal drip as causes of a chronic headache and cough. Coitus cephalgia is not uncommon.

Examination: The candidate will need to demonstrate the ability to undertake focused examination to rule out any focal neurology (including checking plantar response, a brief cranial nerve examination for FAST symptoms), temporal arteritis as well as fundoscopy to rule out hypertensive retinopathy. In a patient with suspected OSA a thyroid examination may also be useful as well as asking for vital signs. A focused cardiorespiratory examination might be useful to rule out cor pulmonale.

Discussion: Complications of sleep apnoea include pulmonary hypertension, hypercapnic respiratory failure, hypertension (an independent risk factor). Investigations include starting off with a simple scoring system like the Epworth sleepiness scale and the STOPBANG score. Overnight pulse oximetry can be used as the first line investigation although polysomnography is ideal and monitors SO_2, ECG, airflow, and abdominal wall movements and this is diagnostic if one has ≥15 apnoeic events during 1 hour of sleep.

Management: Multidisciplinary approach. Patient education. Lifestyle modifications including weight loss, avoidance of alcohol and tobacco. Mandibular assist devices and Continuous Positive Airway Pressure (CPAP). Patient must be advised not to drive until symptoms are adequately controlled and if this cannot be achieved within 3 months the DVLA must be informed.

Differential diagnoses of headaches include.

	Acute	Subacute/Chronic
Single episode	• Subarachnoid haemorrhage • Acute meningitis and encephalitis • Vasodilators such as Nitrates and Phosphodiesterase 5 inhibitors (Sildenafil, Tadalafil etc.) • Acute Angle Closure Glaucoma	• Infections (tuberculosis, meningitis, intracranial abscess) • Raised intracranial pressures (ICSOL, hydrocephalus) • Idiopathic intracranial hypertension • Giant cell arteritis
Recurrent	• Migraines • Cluster headache • Trigeminal neuralgia • Post herpetic neuralgia • Sinusitis • Glaucoma • Coitus cephalgia	• Tension headaches • Cervical spondylitis • Medication overuse headache (common culprits include contraceptive pills, NSAIDs and opioids)

Case 2: Pleuritic Chest Pain

Briefing for examinee: You are on call and have been referred a patient by the GP with pleuritic chest pain.

Briefing for patient: You are a 73-year-old male. You have just come back from holiday in Spain. On the flight back, you developed a right sided chest pain worse on coughing and breathing in. You have developed a temperature and have been coughing up sputum which is blood stained. There is no pain in your calves. You have previously had a clot on your lungs when you were treated with radio/chemotherapy for prostate cancer. However, this is now clear although you continue to be on hormonal therapy with Zoladex (Goserelin). You live with your wife and she suffers with MS. You are her primary carer. You think you might have had another clot on your lungs. Your main concern is that if you are not home tonight there is no one to look after her.

Key Issues: Put PE as a first diagnosis but rule out pneumonia, especially in view of recent travel to Spain. Identify the risk factors for PE, including previous COVID 19 exposure.

A focused cardiorespiratory examination looking to demonstrate features of respiratory failure/cor pulmonale is useful. Do not forget to examine the calves for evidence of deep vein thromboses. Look for scars, lymphadenopathy, radiation tattoos and palpable masses suggesting an underlying malignant aetiology. Please review relevant sections regarding examination technique.

Plan for further investigation if CXR is normal including CTPA. Make plans for further investigation to rule out return of malignancy. Choice and duration of anticoagulation are important taking into account patient's renal function, lifestyle and falls risk. Highlight how to use Well's score. In this case, depending on patient's age and the fact that PE is the most likely diagnosis, this will be high, and a D Dimer should not be done.

The air travel from Spain could be a provoking factor but as this is the second episode and malignancy are not ruled out, lifelong anticoagulation with LMWH may be needed. In terms of addressing the patient's concerns about returning home, one must look at his oxygen requirements and PESI (Pulmonary Embolism Severity Index) score. If the patient is haemodynamically stable, does not need oxygen and the PESI score is low, the patient could be discharged on therapeutic LMWH and further investigations done as an outpatient. On the other hand, if the PESI score is moderate/high risk or the patient needs oxygen, he will have to be kept in as an inpatient and alternate means might need to be suggested, for someone to look after patient's wife. A patient who is haemodynamically unstable will need to be considered for thrombolysis.

Discussion: The examiner might ask you what the relevant findings on clinical examination would be and these include hypotension, tachypnoea, tachycardia, cyanosis, signs of right heart failure/pulmonary hypertension (raised JVP, loud P2, left parasternal heave, dependent oedema) and calf tenderness. Studies have demonstrated that patients with VTE can develop a temperature as part of the inflammatory response. Investigations to include baseline bloods (FBC, U+E, Clotting), ECG (sinus tachycardia, rarely $S_I Q_{III} T_{III}$), CXR, ABG, D Dimer (if Well's score is <4/low risk), CTPA or VQ scan if CTPA unavailable. A Doppler USS could be considered to rule out DVTs.

The following table should help guide your questioning regarding the common and potentially life-threatening causes of chest pain.

Differential diagnoses of central chest pain:

Cardiac:

- Angina: Central; radiation into arms and jaw; precipitated by exertion/stress; relieved by nitrates/rest; typically, 2–10 minutes
- Acute coronary syndrome: Like stable angina but more severe and unrelieved by nitrates or rest; often associated with nausea and vomiting
- Pericarditis: Sharp, stabbing pain worse on movement; preceding history of viral illness

Oesophagus:

- Oesophagitis: Often difficult to differentiate from cardiac pain as it can be relieved by nitrates and is often precipitated by exertion but can be present at other times as well, typically related to meals and often wakes patients up from sleep. Ask about heartburn. Can last for hours.
- Rupture: Usually associated with a preceding history of retching or vomiting

Great vessels:

- Dissection: Classically central chest pain tearing through to the back between shoulder blades; sudden onset; unrelieved by analgesia or nitrates; associated with syncope, bradycardia, new early diastolic murmur of Aortic regurgitation and neurological symptoms

Mediastinum:
Classically retrosternal pain unrelated to respiration or cough unless from the tracheobronchial tree where it has a burning character and is made worse by coughing. A slow growing tumour or lymph node can produce a dull retrosternal ache.
    Common causes of mediastinal pain include the following.

- Mediastinitis
- Malignancies (assoc. with weight loss, haemoptysis)
- Thymoma
- Lymphadenopathy
- Tracheal infections and irritation from fumes/particles

Differential diagnoses of peripheral chest pain:
Pleuritic:

- Infections: History of cough, fever, productive sputum
- Pulmonary infarction and peripheral embolism (can be central as well): classically worse on respiration; associated with dyspnoea, haemoptysis, tachycardia
- Malignancy: Associated with weight loss, cough, haemoptysis
- Pneumothorax: Acute breathlessness; young, thin men or history or chronic bullous lung disease and malignancies as well as connective tissue disorders (Marfan's, Ehler Danlos)
- Connective tissue disorder (history of RA)

Chest wall:

- Musculoskeletal pain: Often worse on movement and associated with chest wall tenderness and trigger points
- Persistent cough/breathlessness: Enquire about common causes of chronic cough — reflux, postnasal drip, drugs including ACE

inhibitors, restrictive lung disorders such as pulmonary fibrosis or obstructive lung disorders such as bronchiectasis and chronic bronchitis
- Post traumatic — fractured ribs
- Infections incl. shingles (dermatomal involvement)
- Tietze's syndrome — Costochondritis — trigger points and chest wall tenderness
- Malignancies (primary lung and pleural cancers as well secondary metastases)

Case 3: Alteration of Bowel Habits

Briefing for examinee: You are on call and have been referred a 38-year-old businessman by the GP with alteration of bowel habits for 6/12 and PR bleeding for 2/52.

Briefing for patient: You are a 38-year-old businessman with a 6-month history of abdominal discomfort and intermittent diarrhoea. There is no history of altered stool or blood in your vomit, swallowing difficulty, indigestion or heartburn. However occasionally you do get abdominal cramps and have lost your appetite. Occasionally you can get very bloated. Now you are opening your bowels about 5–6 times a day, but you can have periods on Loperamide where you go about 3 times a week. There is a feeling of incomplete evacuation at these times. The consistency of your stool can range from liquid to firm pellets or thin ribbon like stools. You have tried to change your diet recently without much success. However, you find that spicy food worsens your symptoms and you have stopped ordering Indian takeaways. Your GP has been treating you for presumed irritable bowel syndrome with Loperamide 2–4 mg as required up to four times a day, but your symptoms have not improved. You have lost one and half stone in weight without trying to in these 6/12. Since the last 2-weeks, you have developed fresh rectal bleeding and symptoms are often worse at night. You were normally fit and well. There is no family history of bowel cancer. You live with your wife and two daughters. Work is stressful and involves a lot of traveling, especially to the Far East. You do not volunteer this information, but when enquired specifically, you admit to having paid for sex during these trips. You have had sex with both women and men. You used to drink quite heavily in the past (1–2 double whiskeys every night and then binge on the weekends drinking up to a bottle of Jack Daniel's and half a bottle of Vodka). You have never smoked but struggle to maintain what is considered a healthy diet. You are here because your GP is worried. Your main concern is that you think you might have bowel cancer.

Key issues: Having a clear set of differential diagnoses here is important. One must delve into a detailed sexual history to extrapolate a diagnosis of AIDS associated diarrhoeal illness. However, it is important to rule out inflammatory bowel disease, coeliac disease and bowel cancers. Be aware of red flag symptoms.

Ischaemic colitis and diverticulitis would be considered in older patients with malignancy becoming more likely with increasing age. Do not forget to offer lifestyle advice including offering help regarding moderation of alcohol intake. If a diagnosis of HIV/AIDS is confirmed, there are ethical issues that can become prevalent such as the patient communicating with his partner.

A gastrointestinal examination particularly looking for features of IBD or gastrointestinal malignancy is expected. Do not forget to offer to perform a rectal examination. Key criteria to differentiate between Crohn's disease and Ulcerative colitis are summarised below including consideration of extraintestinal manifestations.

Discussion: Investigations to include FBC, U+Es, CRP, ESR, LFT, Anti TTG, Faecal Calprotectin, Stool microscopy Culture and Sensitivity incl. Cryptosporidium spores, HIV, Hepatitis B & C serology, CMV serology. The patient will probably also go on to need a CT abdomen pelvis and a flexible sigmoidoscopy with a potential to do a colonoscopy to rule out intraabdominal malignancies.

Aetiology of HIV related diarrhoea:

- Bacteria: Salmonella, Shigella, Campylobacter, Clostridium difficile
- Parasites: Cryptosporidia, Isospora belli, Enterocytozoon, Entamoeba histolytica, Giardia, Microsporidia
- Mycobacteria: Mycobacterium tuberculosis, Mycobacterium avium intracellulare.
- Virus: Cytomegalovirus, Herpes, Adenovirus, Astrovirus and HIV itself (Idiopathic AIDS enteropathy)

Management of HIV related diarrhoea involves general principles such as adequate hydration including replacement of sugars and electrolytes, and if necessary, an elemental diet or nutrient formula with medium chain triglycerides. Lactose and Sorbitol should be avoided. Non-specific medications such as Loperamide and Codeine can be used for symptomatic relief. The underlying cause must be identified and treated.

A summary of the essential knowledge regarding inflammatory bowel diseases for the exam follows.

	Ulcerative colitis	**Crohn's Disease**
Bowel symptoms	• Bloody diarrhoea • Chronic diarrhoea • Abdominal pain	• Abdominal pain (more common) • Diarrhoea (usu. not bloody) • Perianal disease • Fistulas • Strictures
Extraintestinal symptoms	• Sclerosing Cholangitis (PSC)	• Aphthous ulcers • Nephrolithiasis
	Common to both: Dermatological — Erythema nodosum, Pyoderma gangrenosum Rheumatological — Seronegative spondarthritis, Osteoporosis, Sacroiliitis Ophthalmological — Episcleritis, Anterior uveitis	
Endoscopic findings	Continuous inflammation from rectum extending proximally Only colon involved Shallow (mucosal) ulcers	Patchy involvement — skip lesions Can involve any part of the gastrointestinal tract Often involves terminal ileum Deep (full thickness) ulcers
Pathology	• Submucosal Less likely to have granulomas	• Transmural Granulomas more common
Investigations	• Colonoscopy	• Colonoscopy • CT or MR enterography to exclude small bowel disease
Management	• 5 Amino salicylates • Steroids for flares • Immunosuppressants • Biologics	• 5 Amino salicylates (only if colonic involvement) • Immunosuppressants • Biologics
Prognosis	• Approx. 20% lifetime risk of surgery • "Cure" with colectomy • Increased risk of colon cancer (needs surveillance)	• 80% of patients have surgery at some point in their life • Risk of colonic cancer less than UC

Case 4: Syncope

Briefing for examinee: You are an SHO in Internal Medicine at a District General Hospital. A 53-year old Indian gentleman has been brought in by ambulance following a fall associated with transient loss of consciousness. The A&E team have stabilised the patient and are convinced the patient is FAST negative and there is no focal neurology. They have requested you to assess the patient.

Briefing for patient: You are a 53-year old software engineer and moved to the UK 10-years ago. You have been feeling dizzy on standing up from a lying or seated position for the last few months since your doctor readjusted your medications. Today you were feeling very tired and generally unwell at work and decided to call it a day after lunch. Once you reached your driveway and got out of the car you lost consciousness. You recovered after what felt like a few minutes. Your neighbour witnessed the events and called the ambulance.

When asked specifically, you note that there was no warning before the fall today or any associated chest pain, tongue bites, unilateral limb weakness, facial drooping (according to bystanders) or incontinence of urine/stool. You have occasionally suffered with palpitations since your bypass surgery two years ago after a heart attack. You are unsure whether you had palpitations today. These palpitations are irregular and can come on at any time in the day. You used to get these episodes once or twice a year lasting a few minutes but for the last month, they have been more frequent (once or twice a week) lasting up to twenty minutes and are associated with a feeling of being generally unwell and breathless. Other relevant past medical history includes a condition called polymyalgia rheumatica for which you have been on steroids for the last 6 months, hypertension, diabetes mellitus and hypercholesterolaemia.

Your medications are as follows. Please provide this list only if the candidate asks about medications and clarify recent changes as per specific enquiries.

- Ramipril 5 mg OD (increased recently from 2.5 mg OD by your GP; *do not volunteer this information unless enquired about*)
- Bisoprolol 5 mg OD
- Aspirin 75 mg OD
- Prednisolone 4 mg OD (reduced recently by GP from 8 mg)
- Isosorbide Mononitrate MR 20 mg OD

- Metformin 1 g BD
- GTN spray (400 microgrammes) 2 sprays SL PRN for Chest pain

You are intolerant of statins as you get muscle ache with them. There are no other allergies or intolerances. There is a family history of hypertension, diabetes, and heart disease on your father's side (father, uncle and grandfather) but no remarkable history on your mother's side. You are an ex-smoker (having quit after your triple bypass) but smoked 20/day for 30 years prior to that. You drink a glass of red wine with dinner. You drive to work.

There is no history of chest pain, worsening breathlessness on lying flat or at waking up with breathlessness, or ankle swelling. There is no history of cough or associated phlegm, bringing up blood or wheeze. You have no concerns about your bowels or urinary system.

When asked about specific concerns, you would like to know if this is your 'heart playing up'. If the examinee goes on to discuss about driving, express concern as this is important to your profession that you are able to drive. Other than these recent events, you have been in reasonable health and have not lost weight. Your bowels, waterworks, and sleep have been reasonable, but your appetite is low, and you feel generally tired.

Key issues/Problems: This is a difficult but common presentation in the emergency department as there are multiple differential diagnoses and it is important not to miss out on any of them. Given the history a diagnosis of a cardiogenic syncope likely secondary to an arrhythmia is the most likely diagnosis. However, one must ensure that these symptoms are not related to medications, i.e. Iatrogenic (e.g. secondary to significant bradycardia from Beta blockers; postural hypotension secondary to Ramipril and or Nitrates). The patient will likely have an element of hypoadrenalism secondary to exogenous steroid replacement and inadequate replacement might be contributory. It is unlikely given patient's presentations that this was related to poor glycaemic control, but the concept must be entertained. He might even be having significant anaemia secondary to an undiagnosed peptic ulcer in the context of aspirin and prednisolone medication without specific gastro-protective treatment such as proton pump inhibitors. ACEI can worsen renal function further if there is underlying chronic/acute on chronic renal impairment and once again, this could be the first presentation.

Discussion: A thorough cardiovascular and neurological examination is essential associated with key investigations should include relevant bedside investigations (lying and standing blood pressure measurement, a 12 lead ECG, blood glucose, urine dipstick) and lab investigations (including FBC, U+Es, LFTs, CRP, Troponin, 9 am Cortisol, Thyroid function tests). You might want to investigate further with cardiology input with ambulatory/24-hour ECG monitoring and Echocardiogram to rule out structural heart disease. The drugs with the potential of causing postural hypotension might need to be stopped temporarily and reintroduced at a lower dose depending on symptoms and findings of your investigations. The commonest symptomatic arrhythmia is likely to be AF but given this patient's history he might be having scar related life-threatening ventricular arrhythmias. Therefore, inpatient cardiac monitoring and admission are advisable as this would affect management. If any focal neurology were to develop, further imaging would be warranted. The discussion might include questions on management of various arrhythmias, a broad discussion of which is beyond the scope of this book.

Core knowledge review for PACES:

Definition: Transient loss of consciousness resulting in a loss of postural tone caused by period of inadequate cerebral perfusion.

Classification:

- Reflex syncope (previously known as neurally mediated syncope)
- Orthostatic syncope
- Cardiogenic syncope (commonly associated with arrhythmias but also structural cardiopulmonary disease) — characterised by sudden loss of consciousness without warning, which helps differentiate it from other causes which might have prodromal symptoms.

Conditions that mimic syncope:

- Seizures
- Sleep disturbance
- Accidental falls
- Non-epileptic paroxysmal disorders (previously called pseudo-seizures).

These must be specifically enquired about. It is practical to ask for eyewitness accounts and video recordings made by witnesses. Patients who have had multiple episodes will often have relatives and friends who are aware of events and make recordings for the benefit of the patient.

Specifically ask about the patient's position when events happened. A syncope from a sitting position is considered more serious as it is less likely to be a reflex syncope or orthostatic syncope. This is reflected in the DVLA regulations which specifically mention patients with dysrhythmias and structural heart disease as being high risk. Car drivers (Group 1 licence) with a syncope from a standing position due to an identifiable trigger do not have to inform the DVLA if the event happened in a standing position but if it happened in a sitting position, they might not be allowed to drive for 4 weeks. In case of an unexplained syncope they would not be allowed to drive for 6 months. Group 2 licence holders (HGV) may lose their licence for 3 months for a vasovagal syncope or a syncope due to an identifiable cause. If no cause if identified the licence may be revoked for 12 months. The best approach is to tell the patient above but reassure them that you will recheck the up-to-date guidelines (Assessing Fitness to Drive: A guide for Healthcare professionals) and clarify as these are updated regularly by DVLA and subject to change.

Case 5: Deranged Liver Function Tests

Briefing for examinee: You are a senior house officer assisting in hepatology clinic. A 24-year old male was discharged from A&E following a fall — his third admission in 6-months. He was previously fit and well and not on any medications prior to the onset of these symptoms. Upon review with the GP, he was found to have deranged liver function tests. The GP is perplexed as to the cause of his symptoms and blood tests and has referred for further opinion. He has arranged an outpatient USS abdomen, but this is not scheduled to happen until next week. The blood results are attached. The GP's clinical examination of the abdomen was unremarkable other than mild yellowish discolouration of skin and mucous membranes. Your tasks are to take a full history, create a set of differential diagnoses and devise a management plan.

	Value	Normal range		Value	Normal range
Hb	128	130–180 g/L	Na	133	135–145 mmol/L
MCV	81	80–96 fl/L	K	3.9	3.5–5.1 mmol/L
WBC	8.1	4–11 × 10^9/L	Urea	6.1	4–8.2 mmol/L
Neutrophils	6.3	3–5.8 × 10^9/L	Creatinine	83	50–110 μmol/L
Platelets	165	150–400 × 10/L	Total Protein	58	60–83 g/L
Lymphocytes	1.7	1.5–3 × 10^9/L	Albumin	29	35–50 g/L
Prothrombin time	14	11–13 seconds	Bilirubin	60	3–22 μmol/L
INR	1.1		ALT	82	7–56 IU/L
Corrected Ca	2.42	2.2–2.6 mg/dL	ALP	155	44–147 IU/L
Iron	123	60 – 170 mcg/dL	B12	472	190–900 ng/L
Ferritin	101	30–400 ng/mL	Folate	5	2–20 ng/ml
Transferrin saturation	23	15–50%	HbA1c	39	<40 mmol/mol

Briefing for patient: You are a 24-year old chartered accountant of South Asian origin. You were completely fit and well until a year ago when your girlfriend noticed that your mobility and balance were becoming worse. You have had recurrent falls since then and have had to give up riding your bike to work because of the recurrent falls. In the last year there have been three admissions with falls to A&E. On the last occasion, it was noticed that the injuries incurred in the falls took a while longer than usual to stop bleeding. At present you have no issues with your bowels, waterworks or breathing. Only on specific enquiry, reveal that you have noticed that you have a mild tremor at rest. Your father was an alcoholic and this has had a profound effect on your upbringing. You have been a teetotaller your entire life, never smoked and exercised regularly until the recent change in mobility has affected your outdoor activities. There is no family history of note or history of recent travel abroad. Reveal that your parents are first cousins when specifically enquired about. You are sexually active and have been in a steady relationship with your girlfriend for four years and she is concerned about your wellbeing. To the best of your knowledge you have not had unprotected sexual intercourse with anyone else, do not have any tattoos and have never had any needlestick injuries in your life (*Do not volunteer this information unless specifically enquired about*).

Key issues: The key issue is to make the connection that the most likely diagnosis in a young patient with deranged liver function in the hepatitic range associated with mobility issues is likely going to be a metabolic dysfunction, in this case, Wilson's disease, also known as hepatolenticular degeneration.

The history and workup should include a detailed discussion regarding potential causes of chronic liver disease and its complications including the effects of decompensation (Please see Station 1: Section B Case 2 — Chronic Liver Disease). Specifically, in relation to Wilson's disease, and other autosomal recessive conditions, it is important to ask about consanguineous marriages. Although uncommon in the Western world and Indians of Hindu background, marriage between cousins is fairly common practice in Muslim families from the subcontinent. With a growing population of British Asians, this is something physicians need to be aware of.

A brief discussion on Wilson's disease follows.

Supplementary Case: Wilson's Disease

Genetics and Pathophysiology: Autosomal recessive condition associated with a defect on Chromosome 13 resulting in excessive reabsorption of Copper (Cu) from the small intestine and subsequent deposition in the liver, central nervous system (CNS), cornea and kidneys.

Clinical features as per organs affected:

- Liver: Features of Chronic liver disease
- Haemolytic anaemia
- CNS:
  Basal ganglia —
  Extrapyramidal syndrome/Parkinsonism (tremor, rigidity, bradykinesia)
  Cerebellum —
  Ataxia and related symptoms
  Psychiatric symptoms —
  Depression, Anxiety, Psychosis
- Corneal limbus: Kayser-Fleischer rings (golden brown depositions) resulting from Cu deposits in the Descemet's membrane.
- Urinary tract: Renal tubular acidosis.

Investigations: In addition to usual investigations for CLD to rule out more common pathology, the following are specific for Wilson's disease.

- Serum Caeruloplasmin — reduced.
- Serum Copper — elevated/reduced/normal.
- Urinary Copper — elevated.
- Liver biopsy and histopathology — excessive Copper deposition.

Treatment:

- Education.
- Genetic Counselling.
- Copper binders — Penicillamine and Trientine
- Liver transplant for advanced liver cirrhosis.

Case 6: Occupational Asthma

Briefing for examinee: You are a doctor in the respiratory medicine clinic. The GP has asked your opinion on managing a 26-year old man with progressively worsening breathlessness for 6-months. He has moved to the area recently to be close to his girlfriend and was previously fit & well and on no medications. He is allergic to Penicillin.

Briefing for patient: You are 26-years of age. You moved to the area 6-months ago to be close to your girlfriend who works as a nurse in the same hospital. You have been progressively becoming more breathless since moving here. Your symptoms started as a runny nose since you started your new job at a garage. Now you can get very wheezy and breathless. You often have a cough at night, but the cough is not productive of phlegm or blood. There is no chest pain at present but occasionally you suffer with heartburn after a heavy meal.

Only on specific enquiry, you reveal that you spray paint cars at work. You smoke occasionally when you have a drink on the weekends. You only drink a couple of lagers when you're out. There is no one else at home other than your girlfriend. You do not take any regular medications. As a child you had asthma, but you grew out of it as you became older. You do not have any pets. Your breathlessness has been severe enough for you to be off work for the last two weeks. This has improved since then. Your main concern is that you have moved to this part of the country to be with your girlfriend and the breathlessness is progressively getting worse and this is affecting your relationship. You are allergic to Penicillin. There is a family history of asthma.

Key issues: The key features to identify from the history is that this patient is an atopic individual with a history suggestive of occupational asthma on a background of asthma in childhood in addition to smoking. Workers spraying vehicles may be exposed to a chemical called isocyanate, the commonest cause of occupational asthma. Smoking, atopy, allergic rhinitis & childhood asthma are associated with occupational asthma. Gastro-oesophageal reflux is associated with asthma in general and the patient's chronic cough might be postnasal drip, asthma or associated with reflux. It is important to extrapolate and address patient's concerns and effect on his life.

Classically, occupational asthma has also been associated with —

- Additives in flour at bakeries, flour mills and kitchens.
- Farms and agricultural workplaces — grain dust, poultry dust, dust from fungal spores, animal faeces, dander etc.
- Pet shops, zoos, animal laboratories — Fur, dander, saliva.
- Hospitals & healthcare settings — latex, vapour from surgical techniques.

Chemical irritants may also be seen in the following workplaces.

- Woodwork and carpentry workshops — sawdust; dust from sanding/machines.
- Electronics and assembly industries — rosin-based solder flux.
- Engineering and metalworks — vapour from metal working fluids.
- Hairdressing salons — hairdressers' bleach containing persulphate, henna.
- Indoor swimming pools-airborne chloramines.

Familiarise yourself with BTS guidance on management of asthma. Furthermore, the following will be relevant to occupational asthma.

Diagnosis:

History —

- Symptoms improve on days patient not at work/on holiday.
- Worsening symptoms/sleep after work.
- Explore other history of atopy (eczema and allergic rhinitis)

Investigations —

- Skin prick tests to confirm any allergies. Irritants at work as in the above case will not show up on such tests.
- Peak flow diary comparing scores at work/home specifically looking for improvement when off work.
- 'Challenge test' to identify triggers. Only done in specialist centres.
- Eosinophil count on an FBC or serum IgE may also be suggestive.

Treatment — Avoidance of triggers and relevant preventer and reliever inhalers. Patient needs to be addressed in a multidisciplinary approach with advice on patient education which is critical. Do not forget the importance of smoking cessation, vaccinations and occupational therapy in these cases.

Patient education will involve discussions potentially regarding loss of employment if the employer is unable to arrange change in specific job roles. The priority is to highlight that persistent exposure to agents causing occupational asthma can lead to long term asthma, even after quitting the relevant job and life-threatening asthma attacks. You will need to demonstrate empathy and support for the patient during this consultation.

As per Health and Safety at Work Act 1974, the employer must minimise exposure to hazardous substances at the workplace and arrange relevant investigations including a breathing test at the start of employment in jobs where this a risk of occupational asthma. It is also the employer's responsibility to inform the Health and Safety Executive (HSE) if an employee develops occupational asthma. The patient may be able to get Industrial Injuries Disablement Benefits.

Connective Tissue Disorders & Vasculitides — The 2W2P Method

The common cases in the exam are rheumatoid arthritis (the main differential diagnosis of which is psoriatic arthritis), the seronegative spondarthritides (in particular, ankylosing spondylitis), systemic sclerosis and systemic lupus erythematosus. The systemic vasculitides are challenging diagnoses and it is important that you have them on your mind especially if there are associated symptoms of peripheral neuropathy including cranial nerve lesions.

Before we move on to the individual cases, we shall attempt to provide the Two Weeks to PACES (2W2P) approach which can be used when a connective tissue disease/vasculitis is in question. Most patients will present with arthritis. As history & examination must proceed simultaneously, this can be slightly challenging and therefore must be mastered with practice. During the history or examination, if there is a clinical feature suggestive of a disease, inquire and actively look for the other features.

Some useful mnemonics follow. With the connective tissue disorders and vasculitides, be guided by your clinical history but at the same time follow the same pattern with your examination (from general inspection — posture — hands.... Spine, heart, lungs, abdomen) as guided by the 2W2P method to ensure you don't miss anything as often there is significant overlap.

American College of Rheumatology Criteria for Diagnosis of RA 1988: MSH3NFR6

- Morning stiffness >1 h
- Symmetrical arthritis
- Hand joints involvement
- ≥3 joint groups involved
- Rheumatoid Nodules
- Rheumatoid Factor positive
- Radiological changes
- ≥4 or more of the above clinical features present for ≥6 weeks.

American College of Rheumatology Criteria for diagnosis of SLE:

"My dear, please order a sandwich right now. He is awake"
4 out of 11 of the following.

- Malar rash
- Discoid rash
- Photosensitivity
- Oral ulcer
- Arthritis
- Serositis
- Renal involvement
- Neurological involvement
- Haematological disease
- Immunological disorders (Anti DS DNA, Anti Sm Antibody)
- ANA positive

Seronegative spondarthritides: PEAR

- Psoriatic arthritis
- Enteropathic arthritis
- Ankylosing spondylitis
- Reactive arthritis

The Two Weeks to Paces Approach to Connective Tissue Disorders	
History	Examination
Introduction; Presenting complaints. Ask about **SOCRATES** for pain & **ODPARA** of symptoms: **O**nset; **D**uration; **P**rogression; **A**ggravating factors; **R**elieving factors & **A**ssociated features: Be guided by the clinical problem and differential diagnoses. **RHEUMATOID ARTHRITIS — MSH3NFR6** Morning stiffness? If yes, duration >1 h? Joints involved? Joint Replacements? Deformities? Nodules (You can ask as well as check). **LUPUS —** Rashes? Photosensitivity? Oral ulcers? Arthritis? Serositis? Waterworks? **SYSTEMIC SCLEROSIS — CREST** Chondrocalcinosis. Raynaud's phenomenon? Swallowing difficulties or heartburn? Hypertension & breathing difficulties. Systemic features. **SERONEGATIVE SPONARTHRITIDES —** think **PEAR** Axial spine involvement; Distal joint involvement Back pain (sacroiliitis). Number of joints (oligoarthritis) Current/History of psoriasis, alteration of bowel habits (IBD) Dry eyes? Dry mouth? Sjogren's syndrome Loss of vision or hearing and another peripheral neuropathy (mononeuritis multiplex). Then finish **3PMAFTOSA** (**P**resenting complaints including previous investigations & treatment, **PMH**, **P**ersonal history, **M**edications, **F**amily history, **A**llergies, **T**ravel **O**ccupation, **S**ocial history, **A**nything else I've missed?). Enquire about <u>mobility, driving, independence with ADLs, housing, stairs, support at home/work.</u>	**Bedside:** Walking aids, orthoses? **Posture & build:** Stooped? (ankylosing spondylitis); Very tall (think Marfan's) **Hands:** - Deformities (RA, Psoriatic arthritis, Jaccoud's arthropathy) - Nail pitting (Psoriatic arthritis). - Sclerodactyly, Nailfold capillary changes, Raynaud's; Digital ulcerations (Scleroderma) - Clubbing (ILD, bronchiectasis) - Function — Pick up a coin or use a key. - Tendon transfer scars in small joints. - Evidence of neurovascular compromise: Feel pulses. Check power (grip, opposition, thumb abduction) and sensation. Rule out common peripheral neuropathies. **Elbows:** - Rheumatoid nodules - Gouty tophi - Patches of psoriasis **Face:** - Malar rash - Telangiectasia & small mouth - Cushingoid facies — long term steroid usage. **Eyes:** - Conjunctival pallor - Uveitis; Episcleritis; Scleritis - Blue sclera - Pupils: Loss of vision in vasculitides **Scalp:** Psoriasis — dandruff. **Behind ears:** Patches of psoriasis; hearing aids (SNHL in Wegener's granulomatosis)

(Continued)

(*Continued*)

The Two Weeks to Paces Approach to Connective Tissue Disorders	
History	Examination
Systems review Heart — Valvular heart disease, CCF Lungs — Pulmonary fibrosis, bronchiectasis Bowels — Alteration of bowel habits Bladder — Renal function affected by CTD/Vasculitides Sleep/Appetite/Weight loss Check **ICE** (Ideas, Concerns, Expectations). **Summarise**, explain your **management plan (investigations/ treatment)**; arrange **follow up**. Offer leaflets & advise to check NHS Choices.	**Skin:** • Joint replacement scars • Thickened skin (does it go above elbow?) • Elastic skin • Bruises and striations from chronic steroid use Midline sternotomy scars of valve replacement **Spine:** C spine stabilisation scars; Stooped posture. Check range of movement: ask patient to look to the right and left and then stand up against a wall (note the distance) and then to try and touch his toes. The seronegative spondarthritides & RA can affect the spine. **Feet:** Usually MTP joints involved in RA, Oedema in PsA **Heart, Lungs:** Evidence of valvular heart disease; valve replacement scars; pericardial rub. Pulmonary fibrosis (late inspiratory crackles); Pleural rub; Dull bases **Abdomen:** Splenomegaly (Felty's syndrome, Lupus); Evidence of renal replacement therapy

Case 7: Deforming Arthritis Involving Small Hand Joints

7A — Rheumatoid Arthritis

History

Introduction; Presenting complaints. Ask about **ODPARA** of symptoms:
 	
- **O**nset
- **D**uration
- **P**rogression
- **A**ggravating factors
- **R**elieving factors
- **A**ssociated features: Be guided by the clinical problem and differential diagnoses. Ask about:
 	
   ✓ Morning stiffness? If yes, duration >1 h?
   ✓ Joints involved? Joint Replacements?
   ✓ Deformities?
   ✓ Nodules (You can ask as well as check).
   ✓ Peripheral neuropathy?
 	
Then finish **3PMAFTOSA** (**P**resenting complaints including previous investigations & treatment, **PMH**, **P**ersonal history, **M**edications, **F**amily history, **A**llergies, **T**ravel, **O**ccupation, **S**ocial history, **A**nything else I've missed?). Enquire about mobility, independence with ADLs, housing, stairs, support at home/work. *Rule out differential diagnoses: Ensure this is not psoriatic arthritis (the main differential diagnosis). Rule out lupus as Jaccoud's arthropathy looks similar but is in fact soft tissue disease using the 2W2P method.*
 	
Systems review
 	
- Heart — Pericarditis
- Lungs — Pulmonary fibrosis, bronchiectasis, Caplan's lung, Obliterative bronchiolitis
- Eyes — Episcleritis, scleritis, dry eyes?
- Genitourinary — Renal function affected by amyloidosis; glomerulonephritis secondary to Gold & Penicillamine; Circinate balanitis
- Haematological — Anaemia is common (tiredness); Felty's syndrome (RA + Splenomegaly + Neutropaenia).
- Check **ICE** (Ideas, Concerns, Expectations). **Summarise**, explain your **management plan** (**investigations/treatment**); arrange **follow up**. Offer leaflets & advise to check the NHS website (https://www.nhs.uk/conditions/rheumatoid-arthritis).

Examination

Inspect the patient from head to toe.
Bedside: Walking aids, orthoses?

Hands:

- Symmetrical deforming polyarthropathy involving small joints of both hands involving metacarpophalangeal and proximal interphalangeal joints. If erythematous, warm, tender (inflamed) consider disease activity. *Distal joints spared.*
- Deformities include: Swan neck, Boutonniere's deformities of fingers; Z deformity of thumbs; Ulnar deviation of MCP joints; dorsal subluxation at the wrists.
- Clubbing (if present think about Pulmonary fibrosis and bronchiectasis)
- Function — Pick up a coin; use a key.
- Evidence of neurovascular compromise: Feel pulses. Check power (grip, opposition, thumb abduction) and sensation; look out for classical peripheral nerve deformities (esp. look for median nerve release scars).
- *Nail pitting & DIP involvement is a sign of psoriatic arthritis.*

Elbows:

- Rheumatoid nodules
- Ensure no patches of psoriasis

Face:

- Cushingoid facies from long term steroid usage.

Eyes:

- Conjunctival pallor
- Episcleritis, Scleritis, Sjogren's syndrome, Keratoconjunctivitis sicca

Scalp: Rule out Psoriatic patches.
Behind ears: Ensure no patches of psoriasis

Skin:
- Joint replacement scars
- Bruises and striations from chronic steroid use

Spine: C spine stabilisation scar, Atlantoaxial subluxation. Usually only cervical spine involved.
Feet: MTP joints involved in RA. *Pitting oedema in psoriatic arthritis (1 out of 5 cases).*
Heart: Pericarditis — pericardial rub
Lungs:
Pulmonary fibrosis; bronchiectasis — Clubbing + crackles
Pleural effusion — stony dull lung bases; reduced air entry.
Abdomen: Splenomegaly (Felty's syndrome)
Others: Peripheral neuropathy, Carpal tunnel syndrome, Caplan's lung.

Investigations

- *FBC* — anaemia
- *Inflammatory markers* (ESR, CRP — esp. for monitoring).
Serum procalcitonin should be considered if there is suspicion of septic arthritis
- *Autoantibodies*
  - ➢ Rheumatoid factor
  - ➢ Anti CCP
  - ➢ ANA
  - ➢ ENA.
- *U+Es* (? renal involvement)
- *LFT & CXR* (prior to Methotrexate therapy and during follow up; also screen for latent TB before biologics)
- *X rays of joints involved*
- *Ophthalmology assessment* if Hydroxychloroquine is being considered.

Management

General measures:
- MDT approach — PT, OT, SW
- Patient education & psychosocial interventions.
- Treatment & regular follow-up by a specialist; check Disease Activity Score (DAS28), EULAR criteria for response to treatment.
- Bone protection & Vaccination.
- Explain that prognosis is poor (50% patients have significant disability in 10 years; 1/3 patients will lose their job within 5 years).

Medical Treatment:
First line treatment:
- **2 DMARDs (Methotrexate & another) + Short term glucocorticoid** started as soon as diagnosis is made for early control of symptoms.
- **Adjuncts: Analgesia & anti-inflammatory medications** (Steroids and NSAIDs monitoring renal function) during flareups.

Second line (TNF — α inhibitors):
- Severe disease (DAS28 >5.1)
- Inadequate response to intensive therapy with a combination of conventional DMARDs.
- Suppliers provide agents as agreed.
- **Ideally given in combination with Methotrexate.**
- Start with the least expensive treatment.

(Continued)

Management
SECOND LINE OPTIONS INCLUDE: **METHOTREXATE + ONE OF:** - **Monoclonal antibodies** (Adalimumab, Infliximab, Certolizumab, Golimumab, Tocilizumab) - **Recombinant soluble TNF receptor** (Etanercept, Abatacept) - **Janus kinase (JAK) inhibitor** (Barcitinib) (moderate to severe disease; approved March'17) - **Adalimumab, Etanercept, Certolizumab pegol, Tocilizumab, Barcitinib** as monotherapy for people who cannot take methotrexate. *The IL-1 receptor antagonist **Anakinra is not recommended** by NICE on the balance of its clinical benefits and cost effectiveness, except in the context of a controlled, long-term clinical study.* ***Inadequate response or intolerance to at least one TNF-α inhibitor in severe RA**: Rituximab (B cell depleting monoclonal antibody) + Methotrexate.* *If unable to have Rituximab, any of the other second line agents patient was not intolerant to can be tried in combination with Methotrexate. Monitor FBC, LFT, and give Folic Acid with Methotrexate therapy. GET A BASELINE X RAY.* *If Methotrexate intolerant, one of Adalimumab, Barcitinib, Certolizumab, Etanercept, & Tocilizumab can be used as monotherapy.* **Surgery:** - persistent pain due to joint damage or other identifiable soft tissue cause - worsening joint function - progressive deformity - persistent localised synovitis.

Sample presentation & worked example: A case of progressive SOB on a background of rheumatoid arthritis.

This 55-year-old female patient presents with progressively worsening breathlessness on a background of a *symmetrical, deforming polyarthritis involving metacarpophalangeal, proximal interphalangeal and knee joints associated with morning stiffness >1 hour for 8 years treated with weekly Methotrexate. Examination reveals clubbing, Swan neck & Boutonniere's deformities of fingers, Z deformity of thumbs, Ulnar deviation at MCP joints & dorsal subluxation of wrist joints with rheumatoid nodules in the elbows. There is evidence of previous surgery to the small joints of the hands and a right knee replacement.*

Examination of the respiratory system revealed a respiratory rate of 16/minute with fine late inspiratory crackles that did not change with coughing. The observations need to be noted including oxygen saturation. There appear to be no other obvious extraarticular manifestations. These features are consistent with a diagnosis of pulmonary fibrosis and

I would like to suggest an aetiology of either rheumatoid arthritis or Methotrexate therapy based on my clinical findings. The main differential diagnosis for the chest findings is bronchiectasis but the crackles were not of a biphasic nature and did not change on coughing. **The chief differential diagnosis is psoriatic arthritis but there were** *no psoriatic patches visible and distal interphalangeal joints & axial spine were preserved*. The disease is well controlled at present as there is no evidence of active inflammation. The patient's functional status has been affected as evidenced by her having to take time off work, struggles with activities of daily living and her main concern today was difficulty in coping with stairs due to breathlessness. She lives with her eighty-year-old mother and is her primary carer but in her present condition she is struggling to look after herself and her mother.

How would you investigate this patient?

I would proceed to review her observations including oxygen saturations & respiratory rate and arrange relevant investigations including *FBC, inflammatory markers, LFT and U+Es* looking for evidence of complications of rheumatoid arthritis. *Autoantibodies including ANA, ENA, Rheumatoid factor, anti CCP and X rays of joints looking for erosive changes* will be useful to confirm the diagnosis of Rheumatoid arthritis. Arterial blood gas sampling, a CXR (reticulonodular shadowing), Spirometry to differentiate between a restrictive lung defect for pulmonary fibrosis as opposed to an obstructive airway defect such as bronchiectasis and a high-resolution CT can be used to support the diagnosis of pulmonary fibrosis. Bronchoalveolar lavage and CT guided biopsy will be useful in guiding treatment *(Please see Station 1: Case 2B for treatment of pulmonary fibrosis)*.

What is your management strategy?

The disease should be managed in a multidisciplinary approach with early specialist involvement, physiotherapy, occupational therapy and social services to maintain independence with ADLs, patient education and lifestyle modification. Rheumatoid arthritis is managed specifically with analgesia & corticosteroids for flare-ups and disease modifying anti-rheumatoid drugs. Failure to control disease with 2 DMARDs including Methotrexate after 3/12 of therapy warrants the use of biologic agents including TNF-α inhibitors. DAS28 scores, EULAR criteria & CRP are monitored to assess response to

treatment. General measures for pulmonary fibrosis include smoking cessation, annual vaccinations, pulmonary rehabilitation and supplementary oxygen therapy if needed. Methotrexate must be stopped in this case as it could be the offending medication. A trial of steroid therapy may be tried as pulmonary fibrosis secondary to connective tissue disease has good prognosis as it is usually steroid responsive. Antifibrotic agents such as Pirfenidone and Nintedanib have been shown to be beneficial in the ASCEND and INPULSIS 1 & 2 trials respectively.

American College of Rheumatology Criteria for Diagnosis of RA: 1988.

- Morning stiffness >1 h
- Symmetrical arthritis
- Hand joints involvement
- ≥3 joint groups involved
- Rheumatoid Nodules (found in 20–30 % cases; almost exclusively in seropositive patients)
- **Rheumatoid Factor positive**
- **Radiological changes:** Joint erosions; Reduced joint space; Periarticular osteoporosis & Soft tissue swelling.
- ≥4 or more of the above criteria present for ≥**6** weeks.

Although the above criteria have been modified in 2010, they remain quite useful from a PACES perspective as there is a focus on history and examination.

7B — Psoriatic Arthritis

History
Introduction; Presenting complaints. Ask about ODPARA of symptoms: Onset Duration Progression Aggravating factors Relieving factors Associated features: Be guided by the clinical problem and differential diagnoses. Ask about: - Joints involved? Joint Replacements? - Deformities? - Rashes? Scalp involvement? - Axial spine problems? - Back pain (sacroiliitis)? - Vision (anterior uveitis) - PMH of psoriasis, alteration of bowel habits (? Enteropathic arthritis) - Family history is vital Rule out RA: - Morning stiffness? If yes, duration > 1h? - Nodules (You can ask as well as check). ALWAYS finish 3PMAFTOSA (Presenting complaints including previous investigations & treatment, PMH, Personal history, Medications, Family history, Allergies, Travel, Occupation, Social history, Anything else I've missed?). Enquire about mobility, independence with ADLs, housing, stairs, support at home/work. Systems review Heart — Aortic valvular heart disease is strongly associated with psoriasis Lungs — Pulmonary fibrosis Bowels — Alteration of bowel habits (enteropathic arthritis) Bladder — Renal function affected by CTD/Vasculitides Check ICE (Ideas, Concerns, Expectations). Summarise, explain your management plan (investigations/treatment); arrange follow up. Offer leaflets & advise to check relevant websites (https://www.nhs.uk/conditions/psoriatic-arthritis).

Examination
Inspect the patient from head to toe. **Bedside:** Walking aids, orthoses? **Hands: Different phenotypes.** - Asymmetrical oligoarthritis with spinal involvement. - Symmetrical deforming polyarthropathy involving small joints of both hands mainly involving distal interphalangeal joints.   This RA type phenotype can be clinically indistinguishable apart from presence of psoriatic patches with MCP and PIP involvement. If erythematous, warm, tender (inflamed) consider disease activity. - Nail pitting (80% cases), Onycholysis, Leukonychia, Red spots in the lunula, Nail plate crumbling. - Significant periarticular enthesitis, tenosynovitis and dactylitis (sausage digits) - Clubbing (if present think about Pulmonary fibrosis and bronchiectasis) - Function — Pick up a coin; use a key. - Evidence of neurovascular compromise: Feel pulses. Check power (grip, opposition, thumb abduction) and sensation to rule out common peripheral neuropathies (esp. look for median nerve release scars). **Elbows:** - Patches of psoriasis. There is an association of gout with psoriasis. **Face:** - Cushingoid facies from long term steroid usage. **Eyes:** - Uveitis (7%) - Conjunctivitis (20%) **Scalp:** Dry skin/Flakes/Dandruff **Behind ears:** Ensure no patches of psoriasis **Skin:** - Psoriatic plaques (look at inframammary area and umbilicus). - Dry skin, Koebner phenomenon. - Joint replacement scars - Bruises and striations from chronic steroid use. **Spine:** In axial disease, spine is involved. Schober's test may be positive if sacroiliitis. **Heart:** Listen for aortic murmurs. **Lungs:** Pulmonary fibrosis; bronchiectasis — Clubbing + crackles. **Abdomen:** Look for stoma as enteropathic arthritis is a differential for seronegative spondarthritides. **Lower limbs:** Dependent oedema (Found in 21% patients with psoriatic arthritis vs. 5% with other arthritis.

Investigations

- NICE guidance: A negative HLA B27 does not rule out a seronegative spondarthritis.
- No specific laboratory biomarkers.
- Clinical diagnosis.
- **CASPAR criteria to diagnose PsA:** Patients with inflammatory MSK disease (peripheral arthritis, spondylitis, or enthesitis) if they score 3 points out of the following.

    ✓ Skin psoriasis
    Present — 2 points
    Past history — 1 point
    Family history — 1 point
    ✓ Nail lesions (onycholysis, pitting) — 1 point
    ✓ Dactylitis (present or past, documented by a rheumatologist) — 1 point
    ✓ Rheumatoid factor (RF) negative — 1 point
    ✓ X ray evidence of juxta articular new bone formation (distinct from osteophytes) — 1 point

- Rule out other causes:
    Rheumatoid factor +ve 2–10%
    Anti-CCP +ve 8–16%
    Anti-ds DNA +ve 3%
- Inflammatory markers to check activity.
- Radiological changes: terminal phalanx lysis with fluffy periostitis (new bone formation); gross joint destruction; pencil in cup appearance; simultaneous bone joint lysis + ankylosis.

In acute mono/oligoarthritis without clear dermatological disease, crystal arthropathies & septic arthritis might need to be ruled out by synovial fluid analysis.

Management

General measures:
- **MDT approach — PT, OT, SW**
- Patient education & psychosocial interventions.
- Treatment & regular follow-up by a specialist.
- Monitor response with **Psoriatic arthritis response criteria (PsARC)**.
- Bone protection & Vaccination.

Non-biological therapies: NICE recommendations
- **Local corticosteroid injections** as monotherapy for non-progressive monoarthritis.
- For polyarticular, oligoarticular and progressive monoarticular disease, **standard DMARDs** are recommended.
- If a standard DMARD shows inadequate response after 3/12, switch to another DMARD.
- **NSAIDs** as adjunctive treatment to DMARD therapy. If not responding, consider **glucocorticoids** (oral or injections).
- **Addition of a second DMARD** if inadequate control of peripheral spondyloarthritis despite adequate control of extraarticular disease. Patients not on DMARDs were shown to have increased cardiovascular mortality.
- **Targeted synthetic DMARD Apremilast** is recommended in peripheral arthritis with ≥3 tender + ≥3 swollen joints not responding to 2 DMARDs.

(Continued)

Management
Biological DMARDs: NICE Recommendations • ≥3 tender + ≥3 swollen joints not responding to 2 DMARDs. • Usually given alone or with Methotrexate. • Options: First line agents are **Etanercept, Infliximab & Adalimumab. Golimumab and Ustekinumab** can be used based on individual circumstances. **Surgery** Significant effect on quality of life and inadequate response to non-pharmacological and pharmacological measures.

(*Continued*)

PRESENT ACCORDING TO CLINICAL FINDINGS AS THERE ARE DIFFERENT SUBTYPES. A worked example follows.

This 55-year-old male patient presents with progressively worsening asymmetrical, deforming oligoarthritis primarily involving distal interphalangeal joints with relative preservation of metacarpophalangeal & proximal interphalangeal joints associated with morning stiffness <1 hour. Examination reveals tender joints with significant periarticular enthesitis and deformities as well as history of spinal involvement. There are multiple psoriatic plaques with silvery skin flakes and Koebner's phenomenon involving extensor surfaces of elbows, scalp and umbilicus. There were no visible rheumatoid nodules. These features are consistent with a diagnosis of psoriatic arthritis on a background of chronic plaque psoriasis. There were no extraarticular manifestations including aortic valvular heart disease, pulmonary fibrosis and ocular manifestations. Further investigations are guided by patient's history and at present the disease is well controlled with disease modifying anti-rheumatoid drugs. The patient's main concern today was…

Discussion: 5 phenotypes of joint involvement (Moll & Wright) (Mnemonic SODAS):

- Symmetrical polyarthritis with PIP & MCP involvement (indistinguishable from rheumatoid arthritis)
- Asymmetrical Oligoarthritis with DIP involvement
- Distal arthritis (DIP joints) arthritis
- Arthritis mutilans (telescoping of joints with destruction & deformities)
- Spondylitis and/or Sacroiliitis

This polyarticular subtype is commonest and forms the top differential diagnosis of rheumatoid arthritis. Classically, PsA constitutes one of the seronegative spondarthritides (the oligoarticular subtype). In approximately 1 out 5 cases, the arthritis precedes the skin changes (Psoriatic arthritis sine psoriasis) as suggested by distal joint involvement and asymmetric distribution, nail lesions (e.g., pitting or onycholysis), dactylitis and HLA-C*06. Psoriasis is associated with hyperuricaemia and gout and therefore it is not unusual to see gouty tophi. Always FEEL the tophi/nodules. REMEMBER TOPHI ARE HARD AND CALCIFIED, RHEUMATOID NODULES ARE SOFT TISSUE.

Follow the 2W2P method described in the introductory section and be guided by the history and scenario. Ask the patient directly if he was known to suffer from Psoriasis or other skin disorders as well as previous investigations & treatment.

	Rheumatoid Arthritis	**Psoriatic arthritis**
Epidemiology	Female > Male	Male = Female
Clinical Examination	• Symmetrical; usually PIP & MCP involved; DIP joints spared. Usually same joints across digits involved. • Usually only cervical spine involved; remaining spine spared. • No enthesitis • Tenderness before deformity • Polyarthritis • Subcutaneous nodules (20–30%)	• 5 phenotypes; Classically asymmetrical oligoarthritis with axial spine involvement. All joints in digit incl. DIP. • Spinal involvement & sacroiliitis common. • Enthesitis • Usually more tender than RA. Deformity can precede arthritis. • Oligoarthritis • Psoriatic patches • Nail pitting (80%)
Autoimmune screen	70% seropositive (Rh. Factor)	90% seronegative (Rh. Factor)
Genetics	HLA DR4, anti TNF-α activity	HLA B27
X Ray	Joint erosions, Reduced joint space, Periarticular swelling and osteoporosis	Deformity; Pencil in cup appearance with telescoping of joints; juxta articular bone formation.

A Brief Review of Agents Used In RA & PsA For PACES

Anaemia is common in Rheumatoid arthritis and can by megaloblastic (usu. secondary to Methotrexate), normocytic (anaemia of chronic disease) or microcytic (anaemia of chronic disease; associated with gastrointestinal side effects of steroids and NSAIDs). Always provide gastric protection.

Most of the DMARDs can cause bone marrow suppression, skin rashes and haematological abnormalities (neutropaenia, thrombocytopaenia and anaemia) and are hepatotoxic. Monitor FBC, LFTs, CXR and CRP during treatment. Of note are the following.

Standard DMARDs:

- Methotrexate — Pulmonary fibrosis, hepatotoxicity, anaemia (can be megaloblastic due to Folic acid deficiency), hepatotoxicity and chronic liver disease (Monthly FBC, LFT, Baseline CXR).
- Sulphasalazine — Bone marrow suppression, hepatotoxicity, rash (3 monthly FBC, LFT)
- Hydroxychloroquine — Retinopathy (monitor annual visual acuity)
- Penicillamine — Membranous glomerulonephritis, Rashes, Myasthenic syndrome.
- Gold complexes (being used more sparingly) — Membranous glomerulonephritis, Thrombocytopaenia, Rash (Monitor FBC, Creatinine).

Steroids & steroid sparing agents:

- Corticosteroids — Osteoporosis (Always give bone protection).
- Azathioprine — Neutropaenia (FBC monitoring).

Anti TNF-α treatment is contraindicated in:

- Active or latent tuberculosis
- Pregnancy & breast feeding
- Active infections
- History of joint infections (septic arthritis) in the preceding 12-month period
- CCF
- Multiple sclerosis and other demyelinating pathology
- Hypersensitivity reactions

Although the 2019 EULAR/ACR criteria supersede the above 1997 criteria, these remain extremely useful from the perspective of PACES discussion.

Side effects of Anti TNF-α therapy:

- Infections including primary tuberculosis or reactivation of latent tuberculosis
- Haematological abnormalities including malignancies and bone marrow aplasia
- Hypersensitivity reactions
- Worsening of heart failure

Case 8: Ankylosing Spondylosis — The Archetypical Seronegative Spondarthritis

History

Introduction; Presenting complaints. Ask about **ODPARA of symptoms:**
Onset; **D**uration; **P**rogression; **A**ggravating factors; **R**elieving factors & **A**ssociated features: Be guided by the clinical problem and differential diagnoses. Ask specifically about —
 	
• Axial spine involvement — deformities 15–18%; mobility restriction 41%.
• Typically, oligoarthritis.
• Distal joint involvement in extremities [ankles (40 %), hips (36%), knees (29%), shoulders (19%), and sternoclavicular joints (14%)]
• Back pain (sacroiliitis) —
  Age of onset <40 years
  Insidious onset
  Improvement with exercise
  No improvement with rest
  Pain at night (with improvement upon arising)
• Hip pain (25–35% patients) is associated with worse prognosis.
 	
Rule out other seronegative spondarthritides:
Current/History of psoriasis, alteration of bowel habits, recent viral infections.
 	
Then finish **3PMAFTOSA** (**P**resenting complaints including previous investigations & treatment, **PMH**, **P**ersonal history, **M**edications, **F**amily history, **A**llergies, **T**ravel, **O**ccupation, **S**ocial history, **A**nything else I've missed?). Enquire about mobility, independence with ADLs, housing, stairs, support at home/work.
 	
Systems review
 	
• Heart — Valvular heart disease, AV conduction defects
• Lungs — Breathing difficulties (classically apical fibrosis)
• Bowels — Alteration of bowel habits.
• Bladder — Renal dysfunction (8% in one study).
• Poor sleep, fatigue is common.
• Loss of vision (18.6% incidence of anterior uveitis reported in one study).
 	
Check **ICE** (Ideas, Concerns, Expectations).
 	
Summarise, explain your **management plan (investigations/treatment)**; arrange **follow up**. Offer leaflets & advise to check relevant websites such as https://www.nhs.uk/conditions/ankylosing-spondylitis and https://nass.co.uk (National Axial Spondylosis Society).

Examination

Bedside: Male patients (approx. 70%); Walking aids

Posture & build: Stooped question mark posture (fused spine; hyperkyphosis; loss of lumbar lordosis)

Hands:

- Up to 50% patients with axial arthritis will have concurrent distal joint arthritis and deformities. Ensure no overlap with other seronegative disease.
- Dactylitis (6% cases); Enthesitis.
- Clubbing (ILD)
- Function — Pick up a coin or use a key.
- Evidence of neurovascular compromise: Feel pulses. Check power (grip, opposition, thumb abduction) and sensation.
- Ensure no nail pitting (Psoriatic arthritis).

Elbows: Ensure no patches of psoriasis

Eyes: Anterior uveitis.

Skin:

- Joint replacement scars
- Bruises and striations from chronic steroid use; Midline sternotomy scars of valve replacement; Stomas (? enteropathic arthritis).
- Ensure no psoriatic patches.

Spine: Posture already noted. *Kyphoscoliosis. Scars.*

Check *range of movement*: Ask patient to look to the right and left and then stand up against a wall (occiput-wall distance >5cm).

Stand behind the patient and warn him before checking for *sacroiliac area tenderness*. Then mark two points on the spine, one 10 cm above the other 5 cm below the level of the anterior superior iliac spine. Failure of the distance between these marks to increase to >20 cm on bending over is interpreted as a positive *Schober's test*.

Cardiorespiratory examination: Aortic regurgitation; Prosthetic valve clicks; Pacemaker for AV conduction defects; Apical lung fibrosis.

Abdomen: Protuberant. Ensure no stoma (if present? IBD associated arthritis)

Lower limbs: Achilles tendinitis. If erythema multiforme present, think about inflammatory bowel disease.

Sample presentation: *This young male patient presents with a 2-year history of worsening back pain worse at night that improves on activity associated with reduced spinal mobility and progressive fatigue. On examination, he has a stooped 'question mark' posture with limited range of movement of the spine, increased occiput-wall distance >5 cm and a* positive Schober's test with tenderness over sacral region. The patient mentions asymmetrical involvement of ankle and hip joints as well. These features are consistent with ankylosing spondylitis. The other seronegative oligoarthritides are unlikely in absence of any features of dermatological or inflammatory bowel disease. There were no obvious complications such as anterior uveitis and I did not hear any regurgitant aortic murmurs in the heart. There were no fine inspiratory crackles in the lungs suggestive of apical fibrosis. I would like to enquire further about Achilles tendinitis. I would proceed to order blood tests including inflammatory markers & HLA B27 as well as radiological investigation of the spine to confirm my diagnosis.

The patient's main concern was how the disease would affect his employment status and I have reassured him that with treatment most ankylosing spondylitis patients with mild disease are able to remain fully functional and capable of working well in to their fifties. However, a small minority of patients can develop severe skeletal restrictions and extra-articular manifestations.

Investigations	Management
• Clinical & radiological diagnosis. • HLA B27 +ve in 90% cases. • Other laboratory markers are nonspecific. • Raised inflammatory markers (ESR, CRP) in 70% cases.	**General measures:** • **MDT approach — Physiotherapy, OT, SW** • Patient education & psychosocial interventions. • Treatment & regular follow-up by a specialist. • Monitor response with Bath Ankylosing Spondylitis Disease Activity Index (BASDAI) and spinal pain visual analogue scale (VAS). • Bone protection & Vaccination. **Analgesia with NSAIDs:** NICE recommends using the lowest effective dose. If inadequate response to one NSAID after 2–4/52, consider switching to another NSAID. **Anti TNF α therapy:** NICE recommends Adalimumab, Certolizumab, Etanercept, Golimumab and Infliximab in patients intolerant of/ with inadequate response to NSAIDs. Secukinumab is a second line drug when anti TNF α therapy & NSAIDs are inadequate. **Other treatment options available:** **Sulfasalazine** is the only DMARD that is potentially useful. Glucocorticoids are not recommended for long term use. Small trials have shown benefits of **Rituximab, Apremilast and Ustekinumab.** **Total hip arthroplasty** for severe, persistent pain and severe mobility limitations if hip involvement. **Spinal surgery** might be needed in atlantoaxial subluxation.

Case 9: Systemic Connective Tissue Disorders
9A — Systemic Sclerosis

History
Ask about **ODPARA of symptoms: O**nset; **D**uration; **P**rogression; **A**ggravating factors; **R**elieving factors & **A**ssociated features. - *Generally unwell; Fatigue (76%) & weakness (68%); insomnia (66%).* - *Joint stiffness (74%) and arthralgia (67%) — check joints involved.* - *Skin involvement — thickened skin —* **always ask/check if below or above elbow**; *initially pruritus then proceeds to skin pigmentation (47%) & thickening; ulcers at tips of extremities; Calcinosis cutis.* - *Raynaud's phenomenon? Pallor — Acrocyanosis — Reperfusion hyperaemia (White — Blue — Red)* - *Swallowing difficulties or heartburn?* - *Breathing difficulties (interstitial lung disease)* - *Change in your appearance? Ask for old photographs.* - *Dry eyes? Dry mouth? Sjogren's syndrome* - *Mononeuritis multiplex (can manifest as peripheral neuropathy).* - Then finish **3PMAFTOSA** (**P**resenting complaints including previous investigations & treatment, **PMH**, **P**ersonal history, **M**edications (DMARDS, Biologics, Analgesia, PPI), **F**amily history, **A**llergies, **T**ravel, **O**ccupation, **S**ocial history, **A**nything else missed?). *Enquire about mobility, driving, independence with ADLs, housing, stairs, support at home/work.* - Enquire about **Systemic features:** Heart — Hypertension; Systemic sclerosis is associated with risk of pulmonary hypertension; pericarditis (7%) & pericardial effusion; cardiomyopathy secondary to fibrosis; heart failure — diastolic dysfunction (18%) vs. systolic dysfunction (1%); myocarditis; MI; AV conduction defects & dysrhythmias Lungs — Pulmonary fibrosis, Lung cancer (ask about dyspnoea, weight loss, haemoptysis) Bowels — Nausea, Anorexia, Heartburn Genitourinary — Renal failure & crises; 4/5 men have erectile dysfunction; 3/5 women have dyspareunia. **Always check for pregnancy in women of childbearing age as there is a high risk of morbidity & mortality.** Neuromuscular — Peripheral, autonomic & entrapment neuropathies incl. spinal stenosis. - Check **ICE** (Ideas, Concerns, Expectations). - **Summarise**, explain your **management plan (investigations/treatment)**; arrange **follow up**. Offer leaflets & advise to check NHS website (https://www.nhs.uk/conditions/scleroderma) and the Scleroderma and Raynaud's UK website (https://www.sruk.co.uk).

Examination
Bedside: Walking aids, orthoses? **Hands:** - Deformities — Sclerodactyly; initially hands may be puffy & oedematous. - Calcinosis. - Digital ulcers. - Clubbing (ILD, bronchiectasis) - Function — Pick up a coin or use a key. - Evidence of neurovascular compromise: Feel pulses. Check power (grip, opposition, thumb abduction) and sensation. Rule out common peripheral neuropathies (esp. look for median nerve release scars). **Elbows:** *VERY IMPORTANT TO FEEL IF THICKED SKIN EXTENDS ABOVE THE LEVEL OF THE ELBOW.* **Face & scalp:** - Telangiectasia - Small mouth (microstomia) with peri-oral furrowing - Pinched nose - En coupe de sabre (scar down central forehead; literally ') - Alopecia **Eyes:** Strong association with Sjogren's syndrome. **Ears:** Calcinosis; hearing aids (SNHL in Wegener's granulomatosis) **Skin:** - Thickened skin (does it go above elbow?) - Calcinosis cutis **Spine:** Usually spared. **Heart:** Check BP; Signs of heart failure — mainly right heart failure; PPM for AV conduction defects **Lungs:** Pulmonary fibrosis (Fine late inspiratory crackles). **Abdomen:** Evidence of renal replacement therapy. **Feet:** Calcinosis; Infarcts at tips of toes.

Investigations

Haematology & Biochemistry:

- Complete blood count (Anaemia)
- U+E (Renal dysfunction)
- CK (elevated in myositis)
- Urine dipstick (proteinuria; blood)

Serology: 50% sensitive but 99% specific.

- ANA 95% positive
- Anti-centromere antibody (limited cutaneous disease)
- Anti SCI-70 (diffuse disease; associated with systemic fibrosis)
- Anti RNA polymerase III (diffuse disease; increased risk of renal dysfunction & accelerated dermatological changes)
- Serology for differential diagnosis if in doubt, such as RA (Rh. Factor, Anti CCP), SLE (Anti ds DNA), Mixed connective tissue disease (RNP antibodies). ANCA is not associated with Scleroderma.

X Ray of hands:

- Soft tissue calcifications (calcinosis cutis);
- Acro-osteolysis: resorption of the distal phalangeal tufts
- Joint erosions and reduced space
- Demineralisation.

Evidence of complications:

- PFT & HRCT lungs? Restrictive lung disease (ILD)
- Echocardiography? pulmonary hypertension.
- ECG? AV conduction defects.
- Biopsy & histopathology of relevant organs if diagnosis in doubt.

Management

Aims of treatment:
- Symptomatic relief
- Prevent progression
- Treat complications
- Minimise disability

General measures:

- MDT approach — PT, OT, SW
- Patient education & psychosocial interventions.
- Treatment & regular follow-up by a specialist.

Supportive treatment:

- Cosmetic camouflage & LASER for telangiectasia
- Minocycline for infected calcinosis cutis
- Antihistamines for pruritus in early stages

(Continued)

(Continued)

Management
- Gloves & handwarmers for Raynaud's phenomenon. CCB and Prostacyclin may be used. - Dietary modification & PPIs for oesophageal symptoms. - ACEI to prevent hypertensive/renal crises - RRT for end stage renal disease - NSAIDs & short-term glucocorticoids for arthritis. Use with caution if coexisting cardiac or renal disease. - Pulmonary fibrosis is usually steroid responsive. Use steroid sparing agents, antifibrotic therapy, palliative care and long-term oxygen therapy. - Treat heart failure as per ESC guidelines. - Phosphodiesterase 5 inhibitors (Sildenafil) for erectile dysfunction. *Immunosuppressive therapy*: Morphoea: Oral Methotrexate is the most appropriate therapy. Other options include topical treatment with Tacrolimus, Local corticosteroids, Imiquimod & Vitamin D. There might be a role of phototherapy (PUVA). Diffuse cutaneous disease: The choice is between Methotrexate & Mycophenolate mofetil. Methotrexate has no proven role in non-cutaneous disease.

Worked example/Sample presentation:

This 45-year-old coach driver presents with worsening Raynaud's phenomenon in cold weather over the past few months. This is associated with swallowing difficulties, heartburn, generalised fatigue & arthralgia of different joints over the past few years. On examination of hands, I note sclerodactyly, digital ulceration, calcinosis, nailfold capillary changes and thickened skin not extending above the elbow. There is mucocutaneous telangiectasia, microstomia with perioral furrowing and a pinched nose. These features are consistent with a diagnosis of scleroderma and based on skin involvement being limited to below the elbow, I would like to suggest an aetiology of CREST syndrome, a type of limited cutaneous systemic sclerosis.

There were no signs of heart failure or fine late inspiratory crackles of pulmonary fibrosis. There is a positive family history of scleroderma associated with a past medical history of hypertension treated with Ramipril 5 mg OD & gastro-oesophageal reflux disease treated with Omeprazole 20 mg OD. He is also using over the counter Ibuprofen for analgesia and a nasal decongestant for a recent flu. He lives with his wife and is independent with ADLs. His main concern today was prevention of Raynaud's phenomenon as he is out driving in cold weather in the early hours of the morning. I have advised him to use hand warmers/gloves, avoid caffeinated drinks and to stop using the nasal decongestants as these might be contributing factors. I shall see him in clinic in two weeks and if symptoms do not improve, I shall prescribe oral Nifedipine 30 mg/day. I shall also refer him to a rheumatologist for specialist opinion and arrange serological and radiological investigations to confirm my diagnosis.

Discussion: Classification

Classification:

1. **Limited cutaneous Systemic sclerosis** — Thickened skin limited to below elbow and rarely face & neck. Prominent vascular manifestations, including Raynaud phenomenon and telangiectasia. CREST syndrome may be present.
   - Calcinosis cutis
   - Raynaud phenomenon,
   - Oesophageal dysmotility
   - Sclerodactyly
   - Telangiectasia).
2. **Diffuse cutaneous Systemic sclerosis** — Sclerotic skin above the elbow and internal organs involvement.
   Two other phenotypes are known.
3. **Systemic sclerosis sine scleroderma:** No skin sclerosis but vascular & fibrotic features present including Raynaud's phenomenon and other systemic manifestations described in the history.
4. **Morphoea:** Patches of thickened skin.

9B — Systemic Lupus Erythematosus

American College of Rheumatology Criteria for diagnosis of SLE: 4 out of 11 of: *"My dear, please order a sandwich right now. He is awake"* present serially or simultaneously.

- Malar rash
- Discoid rash
- Photosensitivity
- Oral ulcer
- Arthritis
- Serositis (Pleuritis, Pericarditis)
- Renal involvement (Proteinuria >0.5g/24h)
- Neurological involvement (Seizures, Psychosis)
- Haematological disease (Haemolytic anaemia, Leukopenia, Lymphopenia, Thrombocytopaenia)
- Immunological disorders (Anti DS DNA, Anti Sm Antibody, Antiphospholipid Ab)
- ANA positive

History

Step 1: Ask about **ODPARA of symptoms:**
Onset; **D**uration; **P**rogression; **A**ggravating factors; **R**elieving factors & **A**ssociated features. Be guided by clinical problem. The symptoms to ask about:

- Constitutional presentations: Fatigue (80–100%), PUO (50%), Myalgia, Weight loss.
- Symmetrical, migratory poly**arthritis** (90%).
- Skin: **Malar rash** (48–54%), **Discoid Rash**, **Oral ulcers** (27–52%), **Photosensitivity** (41–60%), Hair loss (18–71%), Cold hands — Raynaud's phenomenon (22–71%), Bruise (15–34%).

Step 2: Rule out other systemic arthritis & isolated or coexisting vasculitides:

- **RHEUMATOID ARTHRITIS — MSH3NFR6**
  Morning stiffness & it's duration >1 h? Joints involved? Joint Replacements? Deformities? Nodules
- **SYSTEMIC SCLEROSIS — CREST**
  Chondrocalcinosis. Raynaud's phenomenon? Oesophageal dysmotility — Dysphagia, Dyspepsia? Hypertension; SOB.
- **SERONEGATIVE SPONARTHRITIDES** — Axial spine involvement; Asymmetric oligoarthritis; Distal joint involvement; Back pain (sacroiliitis); Current & past history of psoriasis, alteration of bowel habits
- **VASCULITIC phenomena** — Loss of vision or hearing; other peripheral neuropathy.

Step 3: Finish **3PMAFTOSA** (**P**resenting complaints including previous investigations & treatment, **PMH**, **P**ersonal history, **M**edications — Drug induced lupus, **F**amily history, **A**llergies, **T**ravel, **O**ccupation, **S**ocial history, **A**nything else I've missed?). Enquire about mobility, driving, independence with ADLs, housing, stairs, support at home/work.

Step 4: Systems review (Serositis — Heart, Lungs; Renal, Neurological & Haematological involvement)

- Heart — CP, SOB (Pericarditis, valvular lesions)
- Lungs — SOB (Pleural effusion); Pleural disease in up to 93% autopsies
- Gastrointestinal — Reflux, PUD, Autoimmune and Lupus hepatitis, Pancreatitis (up to 8%), Protein losing enteropathy, Mesenteric vasculitis
- Urogenital — Proteinuria (Lupus nephritis)
- Nervous system — Peripheral neuropathy; Seizures & Psychosis; Anxiety/Depression
- Women of childbearing age — Recurrent loss of pregnancy (with VTE, Migraine, Lupus — Antiphospholipid Ab syndrome)
- Haematological disease — anaemia (tiredness, breathlessness); Neutropaenia (infections); Thrombocytopaenia (Bruises)

Examination

Look at the patient as a whole: Female > male. Afro-Caribbean > Caucasian.

Hands & Forearm:

- Deformities (Jaccoud's arthropathy)
- Symmetrical, migratory polyarthritis.
- Raynaud's phenomenon
- Nailfold infarcts
- Function — Pick up a coin or use a key.
- Evidence of neurovascular compromise.
- Ensure no AV fistulae.
- Ensure no Rheumatoid nodules, gouty tophi, Patches of psoriasis on elbows

Face & Eyes:

- Malar rash
- Cushingoid facies — long term steroid usage.
- Check for mucous membrane ulcers.
- Conjunctival pallor
- Pupils: Loss of vision in vasculitides

Scalp: Non-scarring alopecia (common); scarring alopecia 1/20 cases. Don't forget to look behind ears. Look for patches of psoriasis/hearing aids (SNHL in Wegener's)

Skin:

- Discoid rash
- Joint replacement scars
- Bruises and striations from chronic steroid use
- Livedo reticularis (with Antiphospholipid syndrome)

Spine: Check for scars & range of movement; ask patient to look to the right and left and then stand up against a wall (note the distance) and then do Schober's test. The seronegative spondarthritides & RA can affect the spine but in SLE this is usually preserved.

Lower limbs: Ulcers.

Heart: Pericardial rub, evidence of valvular heart disease — murmurs; valve replacement scars. Ask for BP (hypertension assoc. with renal disease).

Lungs: Dull lung bases — pleural effusion & pulmonary fibrosis (late inspiratory crackles)

Abdomen: Splenomegaly (10%), Hepatomegaly (25%), Evidence of renal replacement therapy (PD catheter, Transplant scar).

Urine dips: Proteinuria, Haematuria (mention).

Investigations
Target end organ damage: - FBC, Coagulation - ESR, CRP - Renal & liver biochemistry - Urinalysis - Blood pressure - Radiography
Serology: - ANA (>98%) - Anti ds DNA (60%) - Rheumatoid factor (25%) - Complement C1q 50%; low C3, C4 - Anti-histone Ab (30–80% positive in drug induced lupus) - U1 RNP (20–30%) - Ribosomal RNP (5–15%) - Anti Ro/SS-A (25–40% Cutaneous lupus; also found in Sjogren's syndrome and congenital heart block) - Anti La/SS-B 10–15% - Cardiolipin (20–40%) — Antiphospholipid Ab

Management

Aims of treatment:

- Symptomatic relief
- Delaying progression & ensuring long term survival
- Minimize target organ damage & side effects of treatment; treatment of complications
- Minimise disability & improve quality of life
- Educate patients about role in management

General measures:

- MDT approach — PT, OT, SW
- Patient education & psychosocial interventions.
- Advise to read up basic information from https://www.nhs.uk/conditions/lupus.
- Treatment & regular follow-up by a specialist.
- Several scoring systems available for monitoring of disease activity (SLE Disease Activity Index; British Isles Lupus Assessment Group Activity Index) and damage (Systemic Lupus International Collaborating Clinics Index)

Supportive treatment:

- Sun protection
- Ensure adequate nutrition
- Advise to quit smoking (increased cardiovascular disease risk)
- Vaccinations.
- Raynaud's phenomenon: Gloves, Calcium channel blockers, Prostacyclin.
- Family planning for women of childbearing age.
  Aspirin should be given from second trimester, esp. with Antiphospholipid syndrome. All pregnancies are high risk should be planned.
- RRT for end stage renal disease

Immunosuppressive therapy & specific management:

- **HYDROXYCHOLORQUINE** or **CHOLOROQUINE** are the drugs of choice.
- In mild disease (skin/joint/mucous membrane disease only), **HYRDOXYCHLOROQUINE** ± NSAIDs &/or short term/low dose (<7.5 mg/day) Prednisolone may be used.
- For moderate lupus (significant but non organ threatening disease), **HYDROXYCHOLOROQUINE with 5–15 mg Prednisolone** in the short term which is tapered off once Hydroxychloroquine begins to take effect. Adjunctive treatment with **AZATHIOPRINE or METHOTREXATE** may be needed.
- **Pulsed METHYL PREDNISOLONE** may be used for severe life-threatening disease for remission induction.
- Other treatment: The monoclonal antibody **BELIMUMAB** has been licensed by FDA whilst RITUXIMAB is used off licence.

Endocrine Disorders in PACES

The two endocrine commonest cases that come up are assessments of thyroid function and acromegaly. We will also aim to cover Cushing's syndrome. However, other disorders such Addison's disease/ Hypoadrenalism, Hypopituitarism and Diabetes Mellitus and the complications associated with it can be expected in the new Clinical consultations station. Ophthalmoscopy relevant to diabetic retinopathy is one of the most important stations to prepare for and will be covered in the Ophthalmology in PACES section that follows.

Case 10: Acromegaly

This case is an end of bed diagnosis. You are expected to pick up the diagnosis from the patient's appearance and proceed accordingly.

History
Introduction; presenting complaints. Ask about **SOCRATES** for headache & **ODPARA** of other symptoms: **O**nset; **D**uration; **P**rogression; **A**ggravating factors; **R**elieving factors & **A**ssociated features: *Tumour related symptoms*: <ul><li>Headache (with pituitary SOLs early morning headaches are common); nausea.</li><li>Anomalies in vision (commonly bitemporal hemianopia)</li><li>Loss of libido; Galactorrhoea in men</li><li>Menstrual disturbance in women</li></ul> *Dysmorphic features*: <ul><li>Change in appearance; ask for old photographs</li><li>Enlarged extremities — Tight fitting rings, bangles etc. Increase in shoe size.</li></ul> *Complications of acromegaly including Systems review.* Endocrine problems: <ul><li>Diabetes — hyperglycaemia; polyuria; polydipsia; tiredness</li><li>Thyroid problems — goitres; features of hyper/hypothyroidism</li></ul> CVS: Hypertension, CCF (SOB, Dependent oedema)   Neurological: Numbness, tingling and pain in median n. distribution   Respiratory system: Snoring; daytime somnolence (? Obstructive sleep apnoea)   MSK: Arthropathy   Excessive sweating.   Then finish **3PMAFTOSA** (**P**resenting complaints including previous investigations & treatment, **PMH**, **P**ersonal history, **M**edications, **F**amily history, **A**llergies, **T**ravel, **O**ccupation, **S**ocial history, **A**nything else I have missed?). Specifically enquire about DM, HTN, IHD and FH.   **Summarise**, explain your **management plan (investigations/treatment)**; arrange **follow up**. Offer leaflets & advise to read up from the NHS website (https://www.nhs.uk/conditions/acromegaly).

Examination
Face: Prognathism (growth of lower jaw); Enlarged lips, nose; Thickened nasolabial sulcus Prominent supraorbital ridges & bossing of skull; Parotid hypertrophy; Loss of oval features of face. Look in the nose for any scars of septorhinoplasty done simultaneously in some cases of trans-sphenoidal surgery. Acne & seborrhoea may be seen. Hirsutism & excessive sweating. **Oral cavity:** Large tongue; Gaps between teeth. **Eyes:** Field of vision; offer to do ophthalmoscopy as some patients might have optic atrophy; 3rd and more rarely 4th & 6th nerve palsy may be present. **Neck/Axilla:** Acanthosis nigricans; Skin tags **Hands:** Enlargement of hands ('spade like'); coarse skin; Wet/ sweaty Check for difference in sensation on lateral and medial sides of each hand and do the following manoeuvres for <u>carpal tunnel syndrome</u>. Tinel's and Phalen's signs. **Chest:** Barrel shaped **Spine:** Dorsal kyphosis **Abdomen:** Organomegaly (liver/spleen) **Quadriceps:** Proximal myopathy (difficulty getting off chairs) **Feet:** Increased size; Thickened plantar tissue

Sample presentation: This 60-year-old lady presents with a history of a persistent early morning headache. On further enquiry she states that friends and colleagues had noticed a change in her appearance and voice. There was no history of lactation, polyuria, polydipsia or hypertension. However, she states that his rings have become tighter and he has noticed enlarged extremities including an increase in shoe size and has put on weight. He had initially had to give up driving because of vision problems but on further enquiry he reveals he has had surgery which improved these symptoms.

On examination, the patient's face exhibits prognathism; enlarged lips, nose and tongue; thickened nasolabial sulcus with prominent supraorbital ridges & bossing of skull. There was evidence of hirsutism & excessive sweating. There were no visual field or cranial nerve defects. The hands and feet were enlarged, and her palms were sweaty with thickened skin. There is no evidence of carpal tunnel syndrome. The patient has a barrel shaped chest but there are no spinal deformities.

These features are consistent with a diagnosis of acromegaly and I would like to examine for any organomegaly and complications of acromegaly including diabetes mellitus and hypertension.

Causes:

1. Growth hormone secreting pituitary adenoma (95%) including as part of Multiple Endocrine Neoplasia syndrome type 1 (Parathyroid adenomas; Pancreatic islet cell tumours and Pituitary tumours; mapped to chromosome 11q13)
2. Ectopic growth hormone releasing hormone production (Carcinoid tumours — bronchial, pancreatic islet cell tumours, adrenal tumours).

Investigations

Biochemistry:
 	
• Growth hormone levels (usually done after exercise)
• Insulin-like growth factor 1 levels: IGF-1 levels are less variable; also raised in pregnancy and puberty
• Oral glucose tolerance test: Failure of growth hormone suppression with 75 g PO glucose.
    False positive tests occur in poorly controlled diabetes mellitus, anorexia nervosa, hypothyroidism, Cushing's
• Check other pituitary hormones & their functional status including ACTH & short Synacthen test; bone profile, PTH, Prolactin, TSH, FT3, FT4, FSH, LH.
• Consider water deprivation test if polyuria and polydipsia not explained by diabetes mellitus
 	
Imaging:
 	
• MRI/CT brain may reveal pituitary adenoma
• CT Thorax/Abdomen to detect an ectopic source of growth hormone
• Echocardiography? cardiomyopathy
• Hand X rays:
    tufting of terminal phalanges
    increased joint spaces
 	
Humphrey's perimetry
 	
Epworth sleepiness scale; Overnight pulse oximetry ± Polysomnography (for sleep apnoea)

Management

General measures:

- MDT approach — PT, OT, SW
- Patient education & psychosocial interventions.
- Treatment & regular follow-up by a specialist.

Specific treatment:

- **Trans-sphenoidal surgery** is the first line treatment in presence of a pituitary macroadenoma.
- FU with IGF 1 and GH levels. If the former is normal and GH levels are <5mU/L, no further treatment is indicated.
- Further treatment with external beam **radiotherapy** and **Somatostatin analogues** (Octreotide or Lantreotide) as injections every few weeks may be considered if symptoms persist after surgery. May be used in patients unfit for surgery as first line agents)
- In presence of elevated prolactin, **a Dopamine agonist** may sometimes be used.
- If above fails, consider the **GH receptor antagonist, Pegvisomant** (proven to reduce IGF1, fasting glucose & fasting insulin by *van der Lely et al., 2001* in 160 patients).

Treatment of complications:

- Weight loss & CPAP for sleep apnoea
- Treatment of CCF and hypertension as per ESC guidelines
- Treatment of diabetes mellitus (lifestyle modification; oral hypoglycaemic agents; insulin)

Case 11: Assessment of Thyroid Function, Goitres

History
Introduction; Presenting complaints. Ask about **ODPARA** of symptoms including **GOITRE** if present: **O**nset; **D**uration; **P**rogression; **A**ggravating factors; **R**elieving factors & **A**ssociated features: Be guided by the clinical problem and differential diagnoses. REMEMBER — Goitres and Grave's disease can be present in EUTHYROID STATE, HYPERTHYROIDISM OR HYPOTHYROIDISM. Pain/Tenderness is a feature of thyroiditis.

Hyperthyroidism	Hypothyroidism
• Loss of weight • Loss of appetite • Diarrhoea • Heat intolerance and diaphoresis • Palpitations • Tremor • Oligomenorrhoea & infertility • Emotional lability	• 'Tired all the time' • Lethargy & weakness; myalgia • Weight gain • Constipation • Hoarseness of voice • Cold intolerance • Menorrhagia • Cognitive impairment

Vision may be affected in Grave's disease.

Then finish **3PMAFTOSA** (**P**resenting complaints including previous investigations & treatment, **PMH**, **P**ersonal history, **M**edications, **F**amily history, **A**llergies, **T**ravel, **O**ccupation, **S**ocial history, **A**nything else I've missed?). Enquire about mobility, driving, independence with ADLs, housing, stairs, support at home/work.

Systems review: A number of these will be covered in the H/o Present Illness
Check **ICE** (Ideas, Concerns, Expectations).
Summarise, explain your **management plan (investigations/treatment)**; arrange **follow up**.
Offer leaflets & advise to check the NHS website
(https://www.nhs.uk/conditions/overactive-thyroid-hyperthyroidism;
https://www.nhs.uk/conditions/underactive-thyroid-hypothyroidism).

Examination

Bedside: General appearance; Evidence of vitiligo?
Build: Overweight (hypothyroid)
Hands: *Start with a handshake feeling the palm, inspect quickly for the following then feel the pulse.*
Hyperthyroidism: Warm, moist hands; Palmar erythema; Tremor. Tachycardia; Irregular pulse.
Hypothyroidism: Bradycardia, Dry skin, Cool peripheries. Evidence of median nerve release? If there is loss of sensation over lateral palm, consider doing Phalen's/Tinel's test. **Thyroid acropachy (clubbing)** & onycholysis in Grave's disease

Face:
   Hyperthyroidism: Anxious, Restless, Fidgety
   Hypothyroidism: 'Peaches & cream' complexion; Round, puffy appearance; double chin; loss of lateral third of eyebrows; thin hair

Eyes: Grave's ophthalmopathy staged as below using the **NOSPECS** acronym. Scars of previous tarsorrhaphy.

- N — Nil signs/symptoms
- O — Only signs (lid retraction/lid lag; ptosis), asymptomatic.
- S — Soft tissue involved (Oedema, chemosis, conjunctivitis)
- P — Proptosis; Exophthalmos >2 cm
- E — Extraocular muscle involvement (complex ophthalmoplegia)
- C — Corneal involvement; keratitis
- S — Sight loss; optic atrophy/nerve compression

Hypothyroidism: Periorbital oedema; Xanthelasmas
Thyroid gland:
Inspection: Scars; Obvious swelling. Ask patient to swallow (Thyroid swelling moves with swallowing); Ask patient to extend tongue (midline swelling that comes up on extending tongue could be a thyroglossal cyst).
Palpation (from behind): Size, Shape, Surface, Consistency, Tenderness, Mobility, Overlying skin.

- Smooth, diffuse goitre — Grave's disease
- Multiple nodules — Multinodular goitre
- Hard — Malignancy

Percussion: Over sternum? retrosternal extension.
If dull, consider checking Pemberton's sign
Auscultation: Bruits. Absence of a carotid pulsation could suggest malignant infiltration.
Cervical lymph nodes
Thighs: Proximal myopathy in hyper/hypothyroidism
Legs/Feet: Pretibial myxoedema ass. with Grave's disease. Brisk jerks in hyperthyroidism while slow relaxation of ankle jerk in hypothyroidism.
Heart, Lungs: Hypothyroidism: Pericardial rub, can rarely lead to cardiac failure (raised JVP, enlarged tender liver, dependent oedema, bibasal crackles).

Sample presentations:

Hyperthyroidism: This 38-year old gentleman presents with weight loss, heat intolerance and bulging eyes. He appears fidgety and restless. Examination reveals warm moist hands with sinus tachycardia and clubbing. There is lid retraction, lid lag and exophthalmos. The visual acuity is normal and there is no evidence of relative afferent pupillary defect. There is a smooth, diffuse non-tender goitre with no local lymphadenopathy. There is no pretibial myxoedema and ankle jerks are brisk. These features are consistent with a diagnosis of Grave's disease with ophthalmopathy and the patient is hyperthyroid.

Hypothyroidism: This 42-year old lady presents with generalised tiredness, weight gain and cold intolerance. She also gives a history of menstrual irregularity and constipation. She is overweight with a 'peaches and orange' complexion and a hoarse voice. There is evidence of sinus bradycardia at a rate of 50/minute. There is loss of lateral third of eyebrows, conjunctival pallor and a previous thyroidectomy scar. There is proximal myopathy with slow relaxation of ankle jerks. She is on Levothyroxine but appears to be inadequately replaced as clinically the patient is hypothyroid.

Causes of hyperthyroidism	Causes of hypothyroidism
1. Grave's disease (76%) — autoimmune hyperthyroidism due to TSH Receptor Antibodies 2. Multinodular goitre (14%) 3. Solitary toxic adenoma (5%) 4. Thyroiditis (3% Subacute thyroiditis; 0.5% Postpartum) 5. Drug (incl. Amiodarone) and Iodine induced thyroiditis 6. Factitious thyrotoxicosis (Exogenous intake; Diagnostic triad of Negligible radioiodine uptake; high T4:T3 ratio & low thyroglobulin) 7. Hashitoxicosis (thyrotoxicosis before hypothyroidism in Hashimoto's disease) 8. Rare: Follicular Ca thyroid, Struma Ovarii, Molar pregnancy & choriocarcinoma	1. Autoimmune disease: Hashimoto's thyroiditis (destructive lymphoid infiltration leading to fibrosis & enlargement) Other autoimmune disease (Grave's disease; Spontaneous atrophy) 2. Iatrogenic (Post thyroidectomy, Radiotherapy and Antithyroid drugs therapy & other drugs including Li, Amiodarone) 3. Transient thyroiditis; Iodine deficiency (rare in the developed world; commonest cause worldwide) 4. Rare: Infiltrative disorders (Amyloid, Sarcoid) & Dyshormonogenesis, Pituitary disorders.

Investigations	Hyperthyroidism	Hypothyroidism
FT3, FT4	↑	↓
TSH	Undetectable	Elevated
TSH Receptor Antibody (TRAb)	80–95% ↑ Grave's disease	10–20% ↑ Autoimmune causes
Thyroid PerOxidase (TPO) Ab	50–80% ↑ Grave's disease 30–40% ↑ Multinodular goitre 30–40% ↑ Transient thyroiditis	90–100% ↑ Autoimmune causes
Thyroglobulin	50–70% ↑ Grave's disease 30–40% ↑ Multinodular goitre 30–40% ↑ Transient thyroiditis	80–90% ↑ Autoimmune causes
Radioiodine scan	High uptake in Grave's disease, Toxic multinodular goitre, Toxic adenoma. Low uptake in De Quervain's thyroiditis	
USS Thyroid	Assessment of nodules/mass	
FNAC	Assessment of nodules/mass	
Nonspecific lab abnormalities	↑ ALT, ALP, γ GT, Bilirubin, Ca^{2+} Glycosuria	↑ CK, AST, LDH, Cholesterol Anaemia; ↓ Na^{+}

Treatment:

Hyperthyroidism	Hypothyroidism
General measures	
MDT approach — PT, OT, SW; Patient education & psychosocial interventions; Treatment & regular follow-up by a specialist.	
Specific treatment	
Propranolol for symptomatic relief. **Antithyroid drugs:** Typically, Carbimazole used as first line agent. Propylthiouracil is the other drug commonly used. Two strategies — 1. Block & Replace 2. Titration — Increase Carbimazole until FT4 in range. Treat for 18/12–1/3rd patients remain euthyroid. If FT4, FT3 ↑ persists options include: • Repeat course of Carbimazole/PTU • Radioiodine therapy • Surgery	• **Replacement of thyroid hormone.** • **Treatment of cause.**

Ophthalmopathy is treated with high dose steroids, and surgical decompression if needed with control of hyperthyroidism.

Radioiodine therapy is contraindicated in presence of ophthalmopathy and smoking should be discouraged. Conventional protective measures should be adopted (Eyedrops and lubrication; Sleep with eyes taped closed). Prism glasses help with diplopia.

Causes of Proximal Myopathy: Mnemonic 6M

Congenital	Acquired
• Muscular dystrophies • Myotonic dystrophy	• Metabolic/Endocrine — Cushing's syndrome, Diabetic amyotrophy, Hyperthyroidism, Osteomalacia • Medications — Steroids, Alcohol • Malignancy — Paraneoplastic syndrome incl. Lambert Eaton myasthenic syndrome • Connective tissue disorders — PolyMyositis, DermatoMyositis, RA

Causes of neck swelling:

Congenital	Acquired
• Thyroglossal cyst • Branchial cyst	• Thyroid swelling (Goitres — Grave's disease, Thyroiditis, Iodine deficiency) • Lymphadenopathy • Vascular causes (Carotid artery aneurysm/tumours; Jugular vein thromboses) • Salivary gland tumours & sialadenitis. • Other benign and malignant tumours, especially neural crest derivatives (Schwannoma, Neurofibromatosis).

Types of thyroid cancers: Mnemonic — **F PALM**

Follicular, Papillary (commonest), Anaplastic, Lymphoma, Medullary.

Case 12: Cushing's Syndrome

History

Introduction; presenting complaints.
Ask about **SOCRATES** for headache & **ODPARA** of other **symptoms: O**nset; **D**uration; **P**rogression; **A**ggravating factors.

Common symptoms: Generalised tiredness, Weight gain, proximal myopathy.
Drug history: Exogenous steroids.
Tumour related symptoms (Cushing's Disease):

- Headache (with pituitary SOLs early morning headaches are common; nausea)
- Anomalies in vision (commonly bitemporal hemianopia)
- Loss of libido; Galactorrhoea in men
- Menstrual disturbance in women

Dysmorphic features:

- Change in appearance; ask for old photographs
- Skin — Poor wound healing, Easy bruising, Acne, Violaceous striae, Hirsutism, Recurrent cellulitis, Hyperpigmentation

Complications:

- *Diabetes* — hyperglycaemia; polyuria; polydipsia
- *CVS* — Hypertension
- *MSK* — Proximal myopathy, Osteoporosis, Avascular necrosis of head of femur (painful hip movements)
- *Eyes* — Cataracts

Exclude pseudo-Cushing's (chronic infection; severe obesity; depression; alcoholism; hypothyroidism).

Then finish **3PMAFTOSA** (**P**resenting complaints including previous investigations & treatment, **PMH**, **P**ersonal history, **M**edications, **F**amily history, **A**llergies, **T**ravel, **O**ccupation, **S**ocial history, **A**nything else I've missed?). Enquire about conditions that might predispose to steroid usage (RA, Obstructive airway disease, Polymyalgia rheumatica etc.)

Summarise, explain your **management plan (investigations/treatment);** arrange **follow up**. Offer leaflets & advise to check NHS website.

Examination
General appearance: Centripetal obesity
Face: Cushingoid facies, Hirsutism, Acne. Avoid the terms 'moon face', 'buffalo hump' and 'lemon on matchstick' appearance as the patient is unlikely to appreciate them.
Eyes: Cataracts; Field of vision? Bitemporal hemianopia with pituitary SOLs
Neck/Axilla: Acanthosis nigricans; Interscapular fat pad
Hands: If pigmentation of skin creases visible, look for adrenalectomy scars as patient might in fact have Nelson's syndrome or ectopic ACTH production
Chest: Gynaecomastia in men
Abdomen: Violaceous abdominal stria; look for bilateral adrenalectomy scars
Quadriceps: Proximal myopathy (difficulty getting off chairs)
Skin: Paper thin skin, bruises, telangiectasia
Feet: Interdigital fungal infections; Onychomycosis (nail fungi)   Then mention you will look for evidence of complications (DM, HTN, Osteoporosis); Steroid responsive conditions (asthma, COPD, RA, SLE, PMR) and Ectopic ACTH secreting conditions (Small cell lung Ca, Carcinoid tumours).

Causes of Cushing's Syndrome:

ACTH Dependent (bilateral adrenal hyperplasia)	ACTH independent
• Cushing's disease (ACTH secreting Pituitary adenoma) • Non-pituitary tumour secreting ACTH (Small cell lung Ca, Carcinoid tumours)	• **Exogenous steroid administration (commonest)** • Tumours of adrenal cortex (Adenomas, Carcinomas)

Diagnostic Investigations:

First line: Demonstrate excess cortisol

- **24-hour free cortisol:** Normal <280 nmol/24h. Values >3 times upper limit of normal confirms Cushing's syndrome and one would proceed to 3rd line tests. Mildly elevated values need further evaluation as these might represent ACTH dependent causes of pseudo-Cushing's with 2nd line investigation.
- **Overnight Dexamethasone suppression test** (1 mg Dexamethasone given at midnight should normally suppress Cortisol measured at 8 am to <50 nmol/l; but in Cushing's syndrome this is not suppressed). Stop artificial oestrogens prior to tests.

Second line: Distinguish Cushing's syndrome from pseudo-Cushing's

- **Low dose dexamethasone suppression test:** Failure to suppress serum cortisol after 0.5 mg Dexamethasone administered QDS for 48 hours helps differentiate true Cushing's from pseudo — Cushing's.

Third line: Localisation of disease

Once a diagnosis of Cushing's syndrome has been confirmed by first line tests, (and pseudo-Cushing's states excluded if needed) the next test to order is a **serum ACTH**. An undetectable ACTH confirms ACTH independent causes and one proceeds to **computed tomography (CT) imaging of the adrenal glands** to rule out any adrenal tumours and ensures there is no history of exogenous steroid administration. If there are no adrenal masses, one might proceed to **adrenal venous sampling or adrenal scintigraphy**.

In presence of raised ACTH, one must distinguish between pituitary and extra-pituitary ACTH production. This can be done by either of the following tests.

- **High dose dexamethasone suppression test**: Failure to suppress serum cortisol after 2 mg Dexamethasone administered QDS for 48 hours suggests extra-pituitary source of ACTH.
- **Corticotropin Releasing Hormone (CRH) test**: 100 microgrammes of CRH increases cortisol production at 120 minutes in pituitary disease but not in extra-pituitary disease.

If cortisol is not suppressed in the High dose Dexamethasone suppression test or increases with CRH, this suggests pituitary disease. Proceed to **pituitary imaging with MRI** and consider **Bilateral inferior petrosal sinus blood sampling**.

Further imaging might involve **CT/MRI of Thorax/Abdomen/Pelvis** for small ACTH secreting tumours.

Other investigations: Test for complications

Serum glucose +/− HbA1c; Ambulatory blood pressure monitoring

Principles of treatment: The chief principle is to reduce cortisol secretion to normal to reverse the clinical manifestations. To achieve this, the secondary objectives include eradication of any tumours, avoiding permanent dependence upon medications and avoiding permanent hormone deficiency.

General Management	Specific Management	Treatment of Complications
- **MDT approach** including **PT, OT, SW**
- Patient education & psychosocial interventions.
- Treatment & regular follow-up by a specialist.	Exogenous Cushing's syndrome — Stop exogenous steroids or taper the dose of steroids if on them for a long term. Endogenous Cushing's syndrome — - Transsphenoidal surgery ± adjuvant radiotherapy for pituitary tumours. - Adrenalectomy for adrenal tumours. - Medical Management — Ketoconazole (1st line), Metyrapone (2nd line)	- Lifestyle modification to treat diabetes & hypertension.
- Anti-diabetic medications.
- Antihypertensive medications.
- Bone protection including Bisphosphonates.
- Cataract surgery.

Dermatology for PACES

The common cases relevant to dermatology in PACES include neurocutaneous disorders such as Neurofibromatosis and Tuberous sclerosis as well as Connective tissue disease such as Pseudoxanthoma elasticum and Ehler Danlos Syndrome. If you have not had an opportunity to do a dermatology job, it is prudent to attend a clinic or two looking at rashes (dermatitis and psoriasis in particular) and dermatological malignancies under the supervision of a dermatologist. Although not common in the exam, it is important to learn about and see cases of diabetic dermopathy, necrobiosis lipoidica and diabetic feet.

Case 13: Neurofibromatosis

End of bed diagnosis — expected to pick up diagnosis from the patient's appearance and proceed accordingly.

History & Examination
• Introduction; Presenting complaints. • Enquire about **SOCRATES** for pain & **ODPARA** of other **symptoms**: **O**nset; **D**uration; **P**rogression; **A**ggravating factors; **R**elieving factors & **A**ssociated features.
Neurofibromatosis Type 1

• Café au lait patches
• Axillary freckling
• Lisch nodules
• Tumours
   — Peripheral neurofibroma
   — CNS tumours (astrocytomas, gliomas)
   — Optic pathway gliomas (usu. in children) affect VA
   — Soft tissue sarcomas
   — GIST
• Neurological manifestations
   — Learning disabilities
   — Seizures
   — Macrocephaly
   — Peripheral neuropathy (palpable nerves)
   — Cardiovascular problems include hypertension (may be secondary to renal/endocrine complications) and cardiomyopathies
• Endocrine: Phaeochromocytoma
• Kidneys: Renal artery stenosis
• Bone abnormalities include short stature, Scoliosis (5%) & Osteoporosis

Neurofibromatosis Type 2		
Neurology	**Eyes**	**Skin**
Bilateral vestibular schwannomas — symptoms include tinnitus, hearing loss and balance disorders. Schwannomas of other cranial nerves Intracranial meningiomas Spinal tumours presenting with pain, muscle weakness and paraesthesia Peripheral neuropathy	Cataracts Epiretinal membranes Retinal hamartomas	Cutaneous tumours Skin plaques Subcutaneous tumours

Then finish **3PMAFTOSA** (**P**resenting complaints including previous investigations & treatment, **PMH**, **P**ersonal history, **M**edications, **F**amily history, **A**llergies, **T**ravel, **O**ccupation, **S**ocial history, **A**nything else I've missed?).

Summarise, explain your **management plan (investigations/treatment)** including Genetic testing, Prenatal testing and Family screening; arrange **follow up** and **genetic counselling**. Offer leaflets & advise to check the NHS website to read up on the condition.

Note: Schwannomatosis is a rare type of neurofibromatosis that presents usually in those aged >20 and manifests as cranial, spinal and peripheral nerves tumours but preserving the vestibulocochlear nerve. The problem lies with the *LZTR1* tumour suppressor gene mutation located on chromosome 22. Symptoms include chronic pain, numbness or weakness and loss of muscle.

Sample presentation: The patient presents with multiple, irregular, cutaneous pigmented nodules. There are multiple neurofibromas on peripheral nerves associated with axillary freckling and Lisch nodules in the eyes. In presence of a positive family history, the most likely diagnosis is neurofibromatosis type 1 but I would like to take further history and arrange relevant CNS imaging and genetic tests to rule out neurofibromatosis type 2.

Diagnostic criteria of NF 1 (AD, NF1 tumour suppressor gene on chromosome 17, Peripheral):

<u>Two of the following</u> —

- ≥6 café-au-lait macules (diameter >5 mm in prepubertal and >15 mm in post pubertal individuals).
- ≥2 neurofibromas of any type or 1 plexiform neurofibroma
- Axillary/Inguinal freckling
- Optic glioma.
- ≥2 Lisch nodules (iris hamartomas).
- Bony lesion (e.g. sphenoid dysplasia or thickening of the long bone cortex) ± pseudoarthrosis
- 1st degree relative with NF1 based on above.

Diagnostic criteria of NF 2 (AD, NF2 tumour suppressor gene on chromosome 22, Central). **One of the following** —

- Bilateral vestibular schwannomas at age <70 years
- Unilateral vestibular schwannoma at age <70 years + 1st degree relative with NF2
- Any 2 of meningioma, non-vestibular schwannoma, neurofibroma, glioma, cerebral calcification, cataract AND one of the following:
  — 1st degree relative with NF2
  — Unilateral vestibular schwannoma AND negative *LZTR1* testing

- Multiple meningiomas AND one of the following
  — Unilateral vestibular schwannoma
  — Any 2 of: non-vestibular schwannoma, neurofibroma, glioma, cerebral calcification, cataract

Constitutional or mosaic pathogenic *NF2* gene mutation from blood tests or identical mutation from two separate tumours in the same individual.

Investigations
• Genetic tests • CNS imaging (CT/MRI) • Biopsy of lesions

Management
General measures: • Treatment & regular follow-up by a specialist. • **MDT approach** — PT, OT, SW; Patient education & psychosocial interventions. • Treatment and regular follow up by a specialist. • Genetic counselling. • Family screening. • Tumour surveillance (annual brain imaging; spinal imaging every 2–3 years) • Manage complications (e.g. antiepileptics for seizures, antihypertensives, academic support for children with learning disabilities etc.)
Specific management: • Surgical resection of cutaneous lesions is not undertaken unless they cause complications such as pain, bleeding, disfigurement or functional impairment. • The most promising targeted therapy for plexiform neurofibromatosis type 1 is with **Selumetinib**, an oral selective mitogen-activated protein kinase (MAPK) kinase (MEK) inhibitor. • Other tumours may be treated with a combination of surgery, chemotherapy or radiotherapy. • Surgery is generally undertaken for vestibular Schwannomas in NF2 if there is a risk of brainstem compression, deterioration of hearing, and/or facial nerve dysfunction. • Successful targeted therapy for acoustic neuromas have been reported with the anti VEG-F monoclonal antibody **Bevaricizumab**.

Case 14: Tuberous Sclerosis

Foot end of bed diagnosis

You may be given some information such as — "this patient has been referred with a rash on their face", or "this patient has had a new diagnosis of epilepsy". Remember the mnemonic **EPILOIA** (EPIlepsy, LOw Intelligence, Adenoma Sebaceum).

History

Any rash should be interrogated with a structured history asking about:
 	
- Where is the lesion?
- How many lesions are there?
- When was it first noticed?
- Was the onset of this skin lesion acute or gradual? Is it spreading?
- Precipitating or relieving factors?
- Previous episodes — when and how long for?
- Medications for this — have they worked or not? Contact history?
- Associated symptoms — pain, itch, bleeding, blistering.
 	
Specific points about epilepsy include:
 	
- Checking there is a pre-ictal, ictal and post-ictal phase.
- Who was witnessed "seizures" and their frequency and nature?
- Abnormal behaviour in complex partial seizures such as lip smacking, chewing or other automatisms
- Abnormal movements
- Brief absences — usually lasting no more than 10 seconds and may be associated with eye fluttering
- Classical (Tonic/clonic) epilepsy — in addition to generalised limb jerking, there may be other features such as tongue-biting and incontinence.
- Precipitating factors, including infection; alcohol/drugs; flashing lights; sleep deprivation; stress; menstruation
- Any predisposing factors including:
  — Family history of epilepsy
  — Previous intra-cranial events (strokes/trauma/infections/space occupying lesions)
  — Birth injury

Examination
- How they were diagnosed? EEG, CT and/or MRI. - Medications for epilepsy Dermatological manifestations: - Angiofibromas (adenoma sebaceum) — red papules in a butterfly distribution over face - Shagreen patches — localised thickening of skin, usually over the lumbosacral region - Ash-leaf patches — areas of hypopigmentation - Subungal fibromas — oval shaped nodule arising from under the nail fold Neurological manifestations: Learning difficulties/mental retardation (50%) & Seizures (80%) Ophthalmic manifestations: Retinal glial hamartomas (phakoma) — white lesion at the back of the globe Abdominal: Palpable kidneys (polycystic kidneys) — look for evidence of renal failure (renal replacement therapy, renal transplant)

Diagnostic criteria are based on clinical manifestations as well as genetic analysis. TSC1 gene is on Chromosome 9 and TSC2 on Chromosome 16 — which code for the protein Tuberin. There is autosomal dominant transmission with variable penetrance.

Investigations	Management
- Genetic tests - CNS imaging (CT/MRI) - Skull radiography — 'railroad calcifications' - USS Abdomen — Renal angiomyolipomas, renal/hepatic/pancreatic cysts - Echocardiogram — exclude cardiac rhabdomyomas.	- MDT Approach — PT, OT, SW - Patient education - Psychosocial interventions - Treatment & regular follow-up by a specialist. - Genetic counselling. - Family screening. - Manage complications (e.g. antiepileptics for seizures, academic support for children with learning disabilities etc.)

Vital Tips for Ophthalmology in PACES

Pupillary disorders are covered in the neurology section. Often candidates are unnecessarily worried about using an ophthalmoscope. The advantage in PACES is that you are entitled to take a history in the stations in which ophthalmoscopy is tested. A few useful tips that can help you get over these reservations follow.

- The trick to familiarise yourself with an ophthalmoscope is to first learn from an expert and then practise on patients. It is an essential skill you will be expected to be apt at as a medical registrar. It might be useful to spend an afternoon in the ophthalmology clinic with a consultant about 4–6 weeks before your examination.
- Always check the patient's visual acuity before thinking about ophthalmoscopy. It might save you the embarrassment of looking in an artificial eye or prepare you for challenges such as an existing cataract.
- Ask the patient what treatments they have had on their eyes and if there are others in the family who have had their vision affected with the same condition. Examinees can confuse retinitis pigmentosa with LASER photocoagulation or drusen. Although it might seem obvious, knowing they have had LASER photocoagulation tells you that they have had neovascularisation and gives you an idea about what you are expecting to see.
- The first step when looking for diabetic retinopathy is to decide whether this is pre-proliferative or proliferative and the single most important determinant is the evidence of neovascularisation. The green light in an ophthalmoscope is particularly useful for looking for microvascular changes in diabetic retinopathy. If you are unsure about whether there is neovascularisation switch to the green light once you can see the retina and the blood vessels will be visible as thin black lines if it is present. The moment you see this, you already know they have proliferative diabetic retinopathy, and you can look for evidence of LASER treatment.

Case 15: Annual Diabetic Review and Diabetic Retinopathy

Briefing for examinee: You are an SHO in endocrinology at a district general hospital. This 44-year-old male diabetic patient has been referred by his GP with poorly controlled diabetes. He has a BMI of 37 and is not tolerant of Metformin due to gastrointestinal side effects. His last HbA1c is 57 mmol/mol. He wants to be referred for bariatric surgery. GP seeks your advice regarding further management. His latest blood results are within normal limits.

Briefing for patient: You are 44 years of age and have always been overweight. You are an HGV driver by profession and struggle to manage a healthy diet or get any regular exercise. You do not want to go on to insulin as you are worried about losing your licence. You have never had any hypoglycaemic episodes whilst driving. You have read on a national tabloid that bariatric surgery can reverse diabetes. Your daughter has done some research on this on the internet and suggested you see your GP as you are clearly overweight and would benefit from surgery. However, you have not really tried to lose weight through exercise and diet. Your comorbidities include high blood pressure and high cholesterol. However, the cholesterol has not been checked in a while as you often work night shifts and struggle to get to your GP appointments or diabetic annual reviews.

You have had some problems with your vision recently. Currently you are on Aspirin 75 mg OD, Atorvastatin 40 mg nocte & Gliclazide 160 mg BD. You normally suffer with dyspepsia and Metformin had made it worse. There is a family history of stroke and diabetes (mother), and your father died from a heart attack at the age of 45 when you were in school. Your elder sister had to have cardiac stents recently. Normally you are mobile and when you are at home you enjoy spending time with your wife and daughters. You gave up smoking 2 years ago at the insistence of family members. Previously smoked 20/day for 25 years.

Key issues/Problems:
As diabetes is a common multisystem disorder, you will need to obtain a systematic and thorough history.

Salient features of the history include:

- Gradual or acute loss of vision
- Floaters
- Details of end-organ involvement

Clinical examination:

- Look for presence of diabetic chart or diabetic foods/juices
- Medications/presence of a glucometer
- Neurological involvement

General examination may reveal

- Finger prick marks
- Presence of diabetic foot
- Evidence of renal replacement therapy

Fundoscopy:

- Signs are shown in the table that follows.
- Remember to differentiate from hypertensive retinopathy.
- Here, there are usually no symptoms
- Clinical features include arteriovenous nipping and arteriolar narrowing and summarised as shown.

Discuss about:

- Poorly controlled Diabetes.
- Obesity — Need to highlight lifestyle modifications and other treatment of diabetes that have not been tried. Can offer other medications before moving on to Insulin including Exenatide if lifestyle and medications are unsuccessful in weight reduction. Highlight importance of trying lifestyle measures and medical management of obesity and T2DM before further assessment of bariatric surgery and review of relevant guidelines.
- Risk of both macrovascular and microvascular complications. Patient should be encouraged to stop smoking. There is no role of antiplatelets without established cardiovascular disease. The need for regular ophthalmology review and footcare should be stressed.
- Reassurance regarding use of insulin in T2DM and update to DVLA guidelines regarding Type 2 (HGV/professional) licences.

Diagnosis	Symptoms	Features	Management
Background retinopathy *Common — caused by microvascular leakage into the retina*	Asymptomatic	Microaneurysms — small swollen red blemish usually seen temporal to the fovea Dot and blot haemorrhages — red blushes scattered across the retina Hard exudates — pale yellow/white patches	Non-urgent referral to eye clinic Annual fundoscopy Manage diabetes and other cardiovascular risk factors such as hypertension and hypercholesterolaemia
Pre-proliferative retinopathy *Uncommon — caused by retinal hypoxia*	Asymptomatic if the macula is spared.	Background changes as above with additional: Cotton wool spots — fluffy white cloudy patches Flame shaped haemorrhages — deeper crimson coloured more linear shaped bleeding Venous dilatation — beading or sausage like segmentation Arteriolar narrowing	Semi-urgent referral to eye clinic Close follow-up to allow detection and treatment of proliferative retinopathy
Proliferative retinopathy *More common in insulin dependent diabetics — caused by retinal hypoxia.*	Asymptomatic if the macula is spared. Can be complicated by vitreous haemorrhage or retinal detachment	As above Neovascularisation around the disc (NVD) — the vessels are flat initially but later are raised and have a pale fibrous component Presence of photocoagulation scars	Urgent referral to eye clinic Argon laser photocoagulation
Maculopathy *Caused by oedema and hard exudates at the macula*	Gradual reduction in acuity, predominantly central vision		As above Argon laser photocoagulation will stabilise acuity in 50% of patients, but may not improve acuity

Clinical Consultations (Stations 2 & 5)

Background

Proliferative

Pre-proliferative

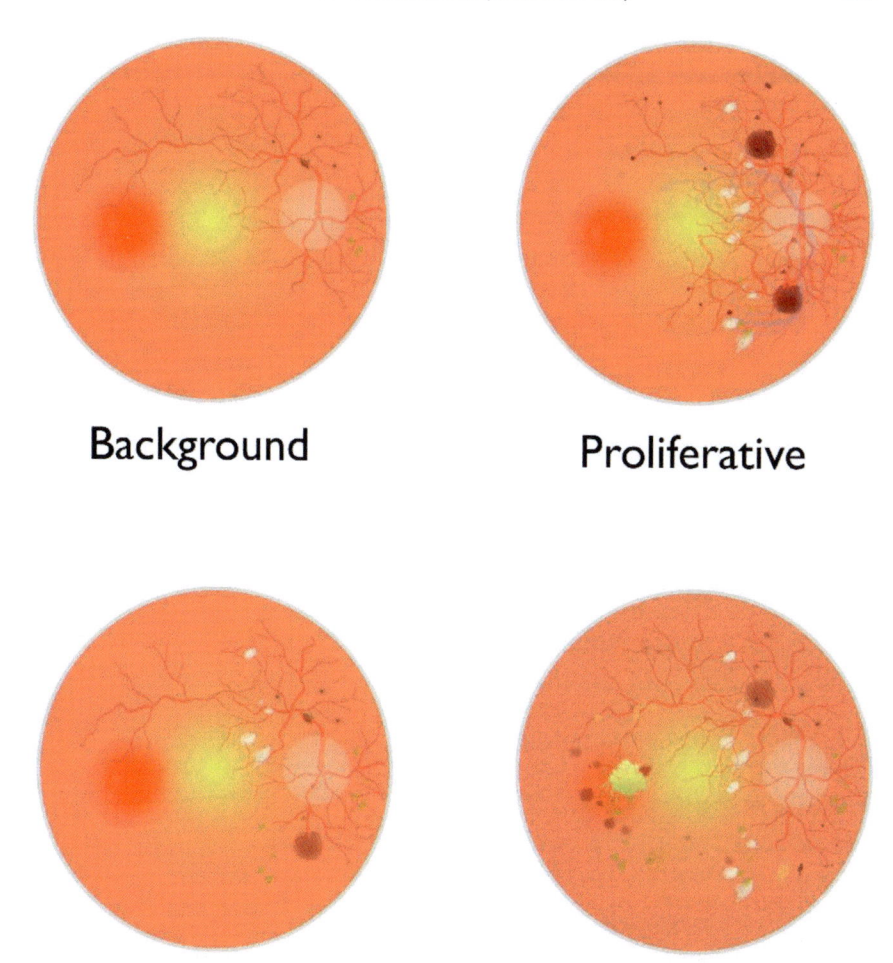

Maculopathy

Discussion:

Diagnosis: Type 2 Diabetes is diagnosed in a symptomatic individual with fasting blood glucose ≥7 mmol/L and ≥11.1 mmol/L on a random sample or after a 75 g OGTT. This must be demonstrated on 2 occasions in an asymptomatic patient. According to WHO, a HbA1c of ≥48 mmol/mol is diagnostic of T2DM but a lower value does not exclude diabetes. HbA1c cannot be used to diagnose diabetes in children, in presence of haemoglobinopathies, haemolytic anaemia, untreated iron deficiency anaemia, CKD, if the patient is on hyperglycaemic agents like steroids and suspected gestational DM.

Management: *"I would like to manage this patient in a multidisciplinary approach with early involvement of specialist physicians, physiotherapy, occupational therapy and rehabilitation services with focus on patient & family education. Specific management involves…".*

Lifestyle modifications: Smoking cessation; Weight loss (5–10%) for overweight individuals; Exercise; Dietary modifications — High fibre, low glycaemic index cards and low-fat dairy products, oily fish.

HbA1c targets should be individualised; checked every 3–6/12 until stable and then monitored every 6/12 aiming for <48 mmol/mol while on lifestyle and Metformin/single agent. The target HbA1c is <53 mmol/mol if patient is on agents that can cause hypoglycaemia or >1 agent.

Choice of antidiabetic medications: Step up if HbA1c >58 mmol/mol.

	Metformin Tolerated	Metformin not Tolerated
Step 1	Metformin	Gliptin/Sulphonylurea/Pioglitazone
Step 2	Add Gliptin/Sulphonylurea/ Pioglitazone/ SGLT-2 inhibitor	Gliptin + pioglitazone Gliptin + sulfonylurea Pioglitazone + sulfonylurea
Step 3	Consider Triple therapy with Metformin + Sulfonylurea + Gliptin/Pioglitazone/SGLT-2 inhibitor OR Metformin + pioglitazone + SGLT-2 inhibitor OR Insulin (along with Metformin)	Insulin
Note:	If triple therapy contraindicated/not tolerated and BMI >35/ or <35 with implications on job if patient on insulin — consider Metformin + Sulfonylurea + GLP –1 mimetic before going to Insulin	

Risk factor modification:

Aim BP <140/90 mmHg unless evidence of end organ damage. Consider ACEI as first line drugs for patients with diabetic nephropathy. However, in patients of Afro — Caribbean origin, A2RBs are the treatment of choice.

Antiplatelets only for patients with existing cardiovascular disease (secondary prevention).

Statins for patients with T1DM, QRISK2 (10-year cardiovascular risk) >10%, eGFR <60 ml/min/m^2 — Use Atorvastatin 20 mg ON which should be increased to 80 mg ON if non-HDL not reduced by ≥40%.

Treat and prevent microvascular disease with strict glycaemic control.

Diabetic neuropathy —

1st line: Duloxetine.

Amitriptyline, gabapentin or pregabalin may also be use if first line treatment fails. Tramadol as 'rescue therapy' for exacerbations and Topical Capsaicin for localised pain.

Gastroparesis — Education, Prokinetic drugs — Metoclopramide, Domperidone or Erythromycin.

DVLA guidance 2016: Whilst going on insulin in the past meant patients could no longer drive professionally, these guidelines have now been changed.

Type 2 licence holders (HGV vehicles, professionals) with insulin treated Type 2 Diabetes can be provided a licence subject to annual review, provided patients have **full** (as opposed to adequate for Type 1) awareness of hypoglycaemia, **no episode** of hypoglycaemia in the preceding 12 months, practises BM monitoring, uses a BM meter which stores 3 months of readings, no disqualifying complications such as visual field defects.

Please see "Assessing Fitness to Drive: A guidance for Medical Professionals" before the exam as these guidelines are subject to change.

Don't forget to ensure you manage all the patient's symptoms, not just their ophthalmic ones, and that you also manage their concerns and expectations.

Awareness of Hypertensive Retinopathy changes is important, as illustrated in the table below:

Grade of Hypertensive Retinopathy	Clinical Features
Stage I	Arteriolar narrowing
Stage II	Irregular calibre of arterioles
Stage III	Cotton wool exudates Dot and blot haemorrhages Flame haemorrhages
Stage IV	Papilloedema

Case 16: Retinitis Pigmentosa

This case will usually present with a history of someone complaining of worsening vision, particularly at night.

History	Examination
Introduction; presenting complaints. Ask about **ODPARA** of **symptoms**: Onset; Duration; Progression; Aggravating factors; Relieving factors & Associated features including other ophthalmic symptoms: • Blurred vision • Altered colour vision • Loss of peripheral vision Finish **3PMAFTOSA**.	Look for obvious signs of blindness such as sticks, dark shades or braille books. The diagnosis will be easily visible on fundoscopy: • There may be an absent red reflex suggestive of cataract • Presence of "Bone Spicule" pigmentation. This is seen to be in the distribution of the retinal veins and spares the macula. • Arteriolar narrowing • Optic atrophy (pale disc)
The remaining history & examination should be focused on identifying and excluding underlying causes as summarised in the following table.	

Management:

- Refer for genetic counselling — most patients are registered blind by the fourth decade
- Aids to assist with poor vision — white stick, braille book, hand railings, etc.
- Support for job applications and training
- Regular ophthalmology follow-up

Cause	Genetics	Clinical Features
Friedrich's ataxia	Autosomal recessive	Cerebellar syndrome Hearing problems Scoliosis Cardiomyopathy (AF/Heart failure) Diabetes mellitus
Refsum's disease	Autosomal recessive	Deafness Cerebellar ataxia Peripheral neuropathy Ichthyosis (dry thickened skin)
Kearns-Sayre syndrome	Mitochondrial inheritance	Ptosis Poor movement of eyes and eyebrows (progressive external ophthalmoplegia) Heart block (look for pacemaker)
Laurence — Moon — Bardet — Biedl syndrome	Autosomal recessive	Learning difficulties Obesity Renal impairment (look for features of renal replacement) Polydactyly Hypogonadism
Usher's syndrome	Autosomal recessive	Congenital Non-progressive sensorineural deafness
Abetalipoproteinaemia	Autosomal recessive	Malabsorption (steatorrhoea, abdominal distension) Scoliosis Developmental delay Spinocerebellar ataxia

SYSTEMIC EXAMINATIONS
(STATIONS 1B, 3A, 3B & 4B)

STATION 1B — RESPIRATORY SYSTEM

Introduction to the Respiratory Examination for Paces

Most candidates will perform the same examination and for the purpose of this book, we shall assume you have honed this skill to pick up relevant signs. A short and succinct 30 second presentation at the end of your examination is the key to success, as it helps differentiate well prepared candidates from unprepared ones. The important negative/positive signs that should be included as a part of every presentation are clubbing, cyanosis, lymphadenopathy, tar staining and venous pressure. We shall provide some brief but important guidelines regarding the examination process.

Look at the patient. Make a note of general physical condition and physical stature. It is especially important to comment if the patient looks comfortable at rest. Do not forget important bedside clues such as medications (inhalers, CREON®), sputum pots or CPAP, NIV machines or nebulisers. If the patient is on oxygen, make a note of how much oxygen the patient is on. These can give you the diagnosis even before you have touched the patient.

Start by asking the patient to take a deep breath in and breath out as quickly as possible and then to cough. If they are expiring for more than six seconds suspect an underlying obstructive pathology. Proceed with hands and make a note of clubbing, tar staining, peripheral cyanosis and asterixis. Take the pulse and respiratory rates. Move to the face (pink puffer/blue bloater i.e. rule out cyanosis). Are there any visible veins? Think about pulmonary hypertension. Feel the trachea.

In the respiratory system, the key clinical findings are on the back. Therefore, we recommend that at this point you sit the patient up and feel for lymph nodes and proceed to examine the back first. Good exposure is paramount as in every other case. **DO NOT MISS SCARS — ACTIVELY LOOK FOR THEM** by looking for subtle faded scars, scars in skin creases and in the axillae as well as any recent dressings over aspiration sites. The importance of scars in this station cannot be overstated and it is easy to miss subtle signs such as radiotherapy tattoos. The presence of the latter gives you a diagnosis of an underlying malignancy.

Inspect (scars/deformities including kyphoscoliosis & depressed chest), palpate (expansion), percuss and auscultate the back on three areas on each side — comparing side to side. Just as one practises listening to heart sounds (discussed in Station 3), the technique to listening to for breath sounds is to practise in this sequence:

1. Inspiration/Expiration. Are the breath sounds vesicular/bronchial/ with prolonged expiration?
2. Is there any wheeze? This is, by definition, expiratory. If you hear an inspiratory sound, this is NOT wheeze but it could be a transmitted upper airway sound or stridor (although beware — stridor really should not come up in your exam).
3. Are there any crackles? If present are they in inspiration or expiration or both? What is their character? Do they change on coughing?
4. Check for vocal fremitus/ whispering pectoriloquy.

Now lay the patient back to 45 degrees and inspect (intercostal recession, pectus excavatum/carinatum, accessory muscle use, scars), palpate (apex beat, left parasternal heave and palpable P2, expansion), percuss (supraclavicular fossa, 3 zones on each side) and auscultate as above. Then look for peripheral oedema, offer to dress the patient and thank them. Then turn to the examiner and mention that to complete the examination you want to check the following — **SPOT X**.

- **Sputum for microscopy, culture & sensitivity**
- **Pulse oximetry**
- **Observation charts**
- **Temperature charts and**
- **Check recent X rays.**

Although not part of the examination, patients with cor pulmonale might have a functional tricuspid regurgitation as well as other signs of right heart failure such as an enlarged, tender liver. If you have time and there are signs of right heart failure, ask for permission to feel the liver and listen to the heart.

Do the above when you are practising on patients in order. Take your time. Learning to listen to breath sounds and heart sounds is like learning to play a musical instrument. You must play every note accurately and in time before you speed up the metronome. Once you get this order right and you've practised enough, you will become slick at this in a few weeks and you will no longer have to worry about what order to do things in. You will just concentrate on picking up the signs.

For all respiratory cases, when asked about management, your first line should always be: *'I would like to manage this patient in a multidisciplinary approach with early involvement of specialist physicians, occupational therapists, physiotherapists and the patient's GP with focus on patient education, lifestyle modification including smoking cessation, annual vaccinations and pulmonary rehabilitation. Specific treatment consists of...".* You would then go on describe medical and surgical treatment options available. The above can be modified for other stations as well but never forget the importance of smoking cessation, pulmonary rehabilitation and vaccinations in this station.

Case 1: The Surgical Chest

1A — Pneumonectomy & Lobectomy

Clinical Examination

The two most important signs to differentiate between the above are position of the trachea and absence/presence of breath sounds.

Classical Signs	Additional Signs Common to Both
• Finger clubbing (might be present) • Cachexia • Thoractomy scar • Reduced expansion on side of scar • Chest wall deformity	• Tar Stained fingernails • Feature of COPD in normal lung • Radiotherapy tattoos • Horner's syndrome • Lymphadenopathy

Pneumonectomy	Upper Lobectomy	Lower/Middle Lobectomy
Trachea **always deviated** towards the side of the scar.	Trachea **may/may not be** deviated towards to the side of the scar.	Trachea is **always central**
Dull percussion notes throughout. Absent vocal/tactile fremitus. Reduced breath sounds throughout although bronchial breathing might be audible in the upper zones.	Percussion notes might be dull at the base if there is an elevated hemidiaphragm. Breath sounds might be normal or absent near the top. The presence of audible breath sounds on the side of the scar helps differentiate from pneumonectomy.	Dull percussion notes with absent breath sounds in lower zones. **Audible breath sounds in upper zone.**

Sample Presentation 1

Mention **SPOT X** (*see introduction*). The patient is comfortable at rest with a respiratory rate of 16/minute. There is a sputum spot and a blue inhaler on the bedside. There is no nicotine staining, raised venous pressure, cyanosis or lymphadenopathy. The trachea is deviated to the left. On inspection, there is a left thoracotomy and the left upper ribs are pulled in. The apex beat is deviated to the left. Expansion is reduced on the same side with dull percussion notes and reduced breath sounds in the left upper zone. There is bronchial breathing in the left upper zone associated with wheeze and biphasic coarse crackles that change with coughing. There is no dependent oedema. These features are consistent with a diagnosis of a left upper lobectomy and an obstructive airway disease. I would like to suggest an aetiology of bronchiectasis in view of the nature of the crackles and presence of clubbing.

Sample Presentation 2

Mention **SPOT X** (*see introduction*). The patient is comfortable at rest with a respiratory rate of 16/minute. The patient looks cachexic and there is evidence of tar staining in the fingers. There is no clubbing, raised venous pressure, cyanosis or lymphadenopathy. The trachea is central. On inspection, there is a radiotherapy tattoo and a left thoracotomy scar. The left lower ribs are pulled in. The apex beat is not deviated. Expansion is reduced on the same side with dull percussion notes and reduced breath sounds in the left lower zone. There are no crackles, wheeze or dependent oedema. These features are consistent with a left lower lobectomy and I would like to suggest an aetiology of an underlying malignant pathology based on the presence of the radiotherapy tattoos, nicotine staining and cachexia.

Sample Presentation 3

Mention **SPOT X** (*see introduction*). The patient is comfortable at rest with a respiratory rate of 16/minute. The patient looks cachexic and there is evidence of tar staining in the fingers. There is no clubbing, raised venous pressure, cyanosis or lymphadenopathy. The trachea is grossly deviated to the right. On inspection, there is a radiotherapy tattoo and a right thoracotomy scar associated with a flattened right chest. The apex beat is deviated to the right. Expansion is reduced on the same side with dull percussion notes and absent breath sounds throughout the right lung field apart from some bronchial breathing over the deviated trachea. The left lung has normal vesicular breath sounds with no crackles or wheeze. There is no dependent oedema. These features are consistent with a right pneumonectomy and I would like to suggest an aetiology of an underlying malignant pathology based on the presence of the radiotherapy tattoos, nicotine staining and cachexia.

Common Discussion Topics

— Differential diagnosis

Pneumonectomy: Malignancy, Bronchiectasis, Tuberculosis
Lobectomy: Malignancy, Bronchiectasis; TB; Lung volume reduction surgery for COPD, lung abscess, empyema thoracis, solitary lung nodules

— Difference between thoracotomy and thoracoplasty
— Types of lung cancer (and para-neoplastic associations)
— Management of Bronchogenic cancer

Investigations	Management
• CXR • Sputum cytology • Pleural fluid cytology • Bronchoscopy & BAL cytology • CT staging • Pulmonary function tests (Pneumonectomy contraindicated if FEV1 <1.2 L)	General: Patient Education, MDT approach, Supportive treatment NSCLC — Surgery — know indications and contraindications — Radical radiotherapy may also be curative. — Platinum based chemotherapy for advanced disease SCLC — Surgery has almost no role — Radiotherapy and chemotherapy may be offered May need a palliative approach including palliative radiotherapy for bone metastases, Rx of Paraneoplastic syndromes See Case 2 regarding treatment of bronchiectasis.

1B — Old TB & Thoracoplasty

Clinical Presentations

- Apical fibrosis (See section on pulmonary fibrosis)
- Thoracoplasty: Surgical removal of upper ribs to collapse the upper lobes.
- Pneumonectomy
- Lobectomy
- Plombage therapy: A "plombe" (fat/wax/Ping-Pong balls/sponges) inserted into the extra-pleural space.
- Phrenic nerve crush: Unilateral diaphragmatic paralysis
- Pleural thickening secondary to recurrent pneumothoraces.

Clinical Examination

Classical Signs of Thoracoplasty	Other Presentations
• Inspection: Thoracotomy scar with evidence of rib resection superiorly & chest wall deformity • Palpation: Reduced expansion on affected side. Trachea & apex beat deviated to side of scar • Percussion: Dull percussion note on affected side • Auscultation: *Breath sounds reduced in upper zones but present in lower zones (helps differentiate from pneumonectomy).* Crackles in the upper zones with bronchial breathing over deviated trachea. Reduced vocal fremitus	• Clinical Features suggestive of apical fibrosis or bronchiectasis • Presence of a supraclavicular fossa scar with reduced expansion, dull percussion notes, reduced vocal fremitus and breath sounds at the base of the affected side is suggestive of a phrenic nerve crush. • A patient who has had plombage therapy might be clinically indistinguishable from a lobectomy.

Common discussion topics: Differential diagnoses, investigations and management.

Differential diagnosis of above to include pleural thickening & effusions, collapse and raised hemidiaphragm.

Investigations	Management
• CXR • Mantoux test • Interferon gamma tests • Sputum cultures (3 early morning sample)/BAL • PFT • HIV testing	• Old TB: History for potential reactivation; Symptomatic management. • Newly diagnosed TB: General supportive measures. Rifampicin & Isoniazid for 6/12 with additional Pyrazinamide and Ethambutol for the first 2/12 intensive phase.

Multidrug resistant (MDR) TB: Resistance to two first line medications. Treatment directed by sensitivity and response to treatment. Usually 3 medications are used until sputum cultures are negative and thereafter 2 drugs continued for 1 to 2 years.

Extensively drug-resistant TB (XDR TB) is a rare type of multidrug-resistant tuberculosis (MDR TB) that is resistant to isoniazid and rifampicin, plus any fluoroquinolone and at least one of three injectable second-line drugs (i.e., amikacin, kanamycin, or capreomycin). Seek specialist advice.

Side effects of first line anti-TB drugs: All the RIPE drugs are potentially hepatotoxic.

- Rifampicin: Reddish tinge to secretions (harmless); Hepatitis; OCP failure (Advise barrier contraception)
- Isoniazid: Peripheral neuropathy (Treat with Pyridoxine), Psychiatric changes, Hepatotoxicity.
- Pyrazinamide: Hepatitis, Hyperuricaemia (gout flare-ups).
- Ethambutol (remember Ethambutol & Eyes both begin with E): Retrobulbar neuritis; Hepatitis.
- Streptomycin: Ototoxicity, Cutaneous reactions.

1C — The Lung Transplantation Patient

Clinical Examination

	Single Lung Transplant	Double Lung Transplant
Signs	Thoracotomy scar Signs of underlying disease on the opposite side.	Clamshell scar
Features of immunomodulatory therapy	• Steroids: Cushingoid facies, back hump, hirsutism, thin bruised skin with purple striae, wasted legs (lemon on matchstick appearance). • Cyclosporin: Gum hypertrophy, Coarse tremor • Tacrolimus: Tremor, Diabetes • Skin cancer removal scars	
Indications	'Dry lung' — Pulmonary fibrosis (note new data suggests double lung transplant shows better long-term outcome), COPD	'Wet lung' — Bronchiectasis, Cystic fibrosis, Pulmonary Hypertension
Management	• MDT approach, • General supportive treatment incl. smoking cessation, flu vaccination, pulmonary rehabilitation • Immunomodulatory therapy & its side effects • Treatment of cause (with single lung transplant) • Treatment of complications (see Liver transplant case) • Ensure follow up	

Problems following transplantation: Remember the mnemonic **GARLIC**

- Graft dysfunction
- Acute or chronic rejection
- Recurrence of original disease
- Lymphoproliferative disease
- Infections and Immunosuppressant drug toxicity
- Cancers and cardiovascular disease

Case 2: Clubbing With Crackles

The differentials include fibrosing alveolitis, bronchiectasis, bronchogenic cancer and chronic lung abscess. The first two are common cases in the exam. We have attempted to present these under one heading because candidates often find it hard to differentiate between cases of clubbing with crackles. We would recommend that the safest way to 'play the game' is to present the most likely diagnosis and give the other as a differential unless there is a sputum pot on the bedside (bronchiectasis), or you are absolutely sure about the nature of the crackles. Often obstructive airway disorders might co-exist or there might be an overlap with cor pulmonale. The key is to show that you are confident with your clinical findings & diagnostic skills and that you DO NOT make up signs (*also the easiest way to fail the exam*).

High yield facts: Common causes of clubbing (Memorise)

- Idiopathic/Familial (commonest)
- Pulmonary: Interstitial lung disease, Suppurative lung diseases (Bronchiectasis, Lung abscess, Empyema), Lung cancer (rare in small cell cancer & mesothelioma), Old stages of pulmonary TB
- Cardiac: Cyanotic congenital heart diseases, Endocarditis
- Gastrointestinal: Chronic liver disease, Inflammatory bowel disease
- Endocrine: Thyroid acropachy

2A — Bronchiectasis

Clinical Examination

Classical Signs	Additional Signs
• Tachypnoea • Finger clubbing • Biphasic coarse crackles that shift with coughing +/– wheeze/squeaks • Symmetrically reduced expansion • Purulent sputum	• Cor pulmonale (raised JVP/RV heave/Palpable P2/ Enlarged tender liver/palpable oedema) • Thoracotomy Scars (old TB/ Lung CA) • Thoracoplasty +/– Midline Sternotomy Scars (Lung +/– Heart transplant) — Cystic Fibrosis (CF) • Rooftop Abdominal Scar (Liver Transplant — CF) • Dextrocardia (Kartagener's)

Sample Presentation

The patient is cachexic and tachypnoeic at a rate of 24/minute. There is evidence of finger clubbing and a sputum pot on the bedside. There is no fingernail tar staining, cyanosis or lymphadenopathy. The trachea is central, and the apex beat is not displaced. The JVP is not elevated. Expansion is symmetrically reduced with normal percussion notes. Breath sounds are vesicular with prolonged expiration and associated with biphasic coarse crackles that shift with coughing and occasional wheeze and squeaks. There is no evidence of cor pulmonale.

The features are consistent with a diagnosis of bronchiectasis and I would like to suggest an aetiology of ... (MENTION DIFFERENTIAL DIAGNOSIS).

Common discussion topics: Causes, Complications, Investigations, Management

Causes
Congenital:
• Cystic fibrosis: small stature; clubbing; crackles; Creon; Porta Cath • Kartagener's syndrome: Bronchiectasis, Dextrocardia, Sinusitis and Azoospermia
Acquired:
• Infections — Tuberculosis, Measles • Recurrent aspiration — GORD, Alcoholics • Connective tissue disorders • Allergic bronchopulmonary aspergillosis • Hypogammaglobulinaemia

Complications: Empyema, Haemoptysis, Cor pulmonale, Pneumothorax, Sinusitis, Pleural effusion, Amyloidosis, Brain abscess

General measures in management of all respiratory patients (memorise): *"I would like to manage this patient in a multidisciplinary approach with early involvement of specialist physicians, occupational therapists, physiotherapists and the patient's GP with focus on patient education, lifestyle modification including smoking cessation, annual vaccinations and pulmonary rehabilitation. Specific treatment consists of ..."*

Investigations	Management
<ul><li>CXR (tramline shadows showing thickened bronchial walls}</li><li>Sputum culture</li><li>O2 saturation ± Arterial blood gas analyses to assess level of hypoxia</li><li>PFT — Obstructive picture (helps differentiate from pulmonary fibrosis)</li><li>HRCT — Tram track lines or signet-ring appearance of a dilated bronchus</li><li>Sweat Sodium Concentration >60mmol/L (for cystic fibrosis)</li></ul>	<ul><li>DON'T FORGET GENERAL MEASURES</li><li>**Regular postural drainage**</li><li>High dose, broad spectrum antibiotics for infections (with anti-pseudomonal cover)</li><li>Long term antibiotic prophylaxis</li><li>Immunisation</li><li>Mucolytics</li><li>Bronchodilators & inhaled corticosteroids</li><li>Surgery (selected cases)</li></ul> **Specific for CF:**<ul><li>Pancreatic enzyme replacement.</li><li>Lung transplant.</li><li>Gene therapy.</li></ul>

Cystic Fibrosis: All you need to know for PACES

Genetics
CFTR gene (Chloride channel) defect; Chromosome 7; deletion of Δ508/Δ508 (commonest mutation) — results in thickened secretions that block luminal structures.
Features
<ul><li>Respiratory: nasal polyps, otitis media, bronchiolitis, bronchiectasis secondary to recurrent pneumonia.</li><li>Gastrointestinal tract: loss of pancreatic exocrine functions — resulting in malabsorption and steatorrhoea, gall stones & secondary biliary cirrhosis, meconium ileus in children, distal intestinal obstruction syndrome (DIOS) in adults.</li><li>Urogenital: Infertility (both in males and females)</li><li>Others: Loss of endocrine function of pancreas, non-invasive arthropathy.</li></ul>
Key Signs
Short stature; clubbing; sputum pot (purulent) & CREON® on the bedside; hyperinflated chest, coarse biphasic crackles that shift on coughing and squeaks/wheeze; Porta Cath® or Hickman lines for antibiotics.
Management
As above

2B — Pulmonary Fibrosis

Clinical Examination

Classical Signs	Additional Signs
• Tachypnoea • Finger clubbing • Symmetrically reduced chest expansion • Bilateral basal fine late inspiratory crackles	May have: • Features of RA/CREST/Ankylosing Spondylitis/other vasculitides • Radiation Marks/Slate-Grey appearance of Amiodarone toxicity • Central cyanosis • Loud P2 and right ventricular heave (if pulmonary hypertension) • "Cushingoid" appearance from steroid therapy • Evidence of cor pulmonale in advanced cases

Sample Presentation

"The patient is tachypnoeic at a rate of 24 breaths/minute and is using ambulatory oxygen therapy. There is clubbing in both hands associated with evidence of connective tissue disease as evidenced by sclerodactyly, flexion deformities and evidence of soft tissue atrophy at the fingertips. The skin is sclerotic and appears smooth, shiny and tight and extends above the elbow. Facial skin has a similar appearance with evidence of telangiectasia. The nose appears to be pinched with restrictive mouth opening.

There is a small scar in the right thorax suggestive of previous lung biopsy. The trachea is central, and the apex beat is not displaced. The venous pressure is elevated and there is a palpable P2 and right ventricular heave. The expansion is reduced symmetrically, and percussion notes are dull at the bases. Breath sounds are vesicular in all areas and associated with fine late inspiratory crackles that do no shift with coughing. There is peripheral oedema up to mid shin. There is no lymphadenopathy, cyanosis or tar staining.

These features are consistent with a diagnosis of pulmonary fibrosis complicated by pulmonary hypertension and cor pulmonale and I would like to suggest an aetiology of systemic sclerosis."

Common Discussion Topics

- Differential diagnoses
- Investigations
- Management

As in the example above, based on your clinical examination, suggest the most likely diagnoses and then mention other differentials as listed in the table that follows.

Aetiology	
Upper Zone (ROAST)	**Lower Zone (ACID)**
• R — Radiation • O — Occupational diseases (except Asbestos) • A — Allergic Reactions (Extrinsic Allergic Alveolitis & ABPA); Ankylosing spondylitis • S — Sarcoidosis • T — Tuberculosis	• A — Asbestosis (All inhaled agents except Asbestos cause upper zone fibrosis). • C — Connective tissue disease (except Ankylosing spondylitis) • I — Idiopathic • D — Drugs (BADMAN — Bleomycin, Adriamycin, Doxorubicin, Methotrexate, Amiodarone, Nitrofurantoin)
Investigations	
• CXR (reticulonodular shadowing) • Spirometry — a restrictive lung defect, i.e. FEV1/FVC > 80% • Arterial blood gas sampling • Autoantibodies: ANA, ENA & Rheumatoid factor • HRCT shows a ground glass appearance • Bronchoalveolar lavage shows a lymphocytic fluid • Open Lung Biopsy	
Management	
• General & supportive management — MDT approach, specialist opinion, PT, OT, patient education, lifestyle modification including smoking cessation, annual vaccinations and pulmonary rehabilitation, supplementary oxygen therapy & palliative care if end of life. • Specific management — Depends on whether this is idiopathic or secondary to another cause. • Stop offending medications & treatment of cause • Immunosuppression with **STEROIDS/STEROID SPARING AGENTS if** there an inflammatory pathology. Better prognosis if steroid responsive. Combination therapy is no longer recommended (PANTHER trial) • **PIRFENIDONE** (ASCEND trial) & **NINTENADIB** (INPULSIS 1 & 2) have been shown to slow progress in idiopathic fibrosis. • If there are no contraindications, a trial of **SILDENAFIL** can be used in advanced IPF with DLCO < 35 %, echocardiographic evidence of RVF. • **LUNG TRANSPLANT**: The ISLHT 2012 trail showed better long-term prognosis with double lung transplant over single lung transplantation. Viable if patient less than 65 years of age + TLCO < 40% predicted and progressive decline in FVC > 15 % in 6/12. • **TREATMENT OF REFLUX** has been shown to improve outcome in IPF.	

Case 3: Dullness At The Lung Bases

3A — Pleural Effusion

Examination Findings

Classical Signs	Additional Signs
On the side of the effusion: • Reduced expansion • 'Stony' Dull percussion notes • Reduced breath sounds • Reduced vocal resonance • There might be bronchial breathing or crackles above the area of dullness	• Cachexia • Aspiration/chest drain marks • Evidence of cause: clubbing, tar staining, lymphadenopathy, previous mastectomy, peripheral oedema (heart failure) • Tracheal deviation to opposite side (with large effusions)

Sample Presentation

To complete my examination, I would like to SPOT X (*see introduction to chapter*). The patient is comfortable at rest. The patient is not cachectic and there is no evidence of clubbing, nicotine staining, asterixis, cyanosis or lymphadenopathy. The venous pressure is not elevated. There are no visible scars. On the right side, the expansion is reduced with stony dull percussion notes and diminished breath sounds. The vocal fremitus is reduced (*helps differentiate from consolidation*). There is no peripheral oedema.

These features are consistent with a diagnosis of pleural effusion. Other differentials include pleural thickening.

Differential diagnosis of a dull lung base: Pleural effusion, Pleural thickening, Consolidation, Collapse, Fibrosis, Elevated hemidiaphragm, Lower lobectomy (if scar present)

Discussion Topics

- Differential diagnoses
- Light's criteria
- Transudative (failures — heart, liver, kidney) versus Exudative effusions (infections, neoplasms, connective tissue disorders)
- Investigations
- Management — General and Specific — according to cause.

Investigations	Light's Criteria
- ABG — assess hypoxia - CXR - USS - Pleural aspirate - CT - Vasculitis screen	An exudate if any of the following: - Pleural fluid protein: serum protein >0.5 - Pleural fluid LDH: serum LDH >0.6 - Pleural fluid LDH >2/3 upper limit of normal serum value

3B — Consolidation

Examination Findings

Classical Signs	Additional Signs
- Tachypnoea - Trachea central - Normal/reduced chest expansion - 'Woody' dull percussion notes - Bronchial breathing or Coarse crackles ± pleural rub - Increased vocal fremitus	- Intravenous cannula (IV Antibiotics) - Sputum pot

Quick Revision

Differentials: Pneumonia, Consolidation with distal neoplasm, Collapse (expect tracheal deviation), Pleural effusion — 'stony dull' percussion notes

Investigations	Management
- CXR - ABG — assess hypoxia - CT chest if diagnosis unclear ± tumour markers - Sputum culture - Urinary antigen for Legionella and Pneumococci - Consider HIV test if typical pneumonia	- Antibiotic therapy is guided by local antimicrobial policy and guidelines. CURB 65 score may be used. - Supplementary oxygen therapy

Case 4: Chronic Obstructive Airway Disease

Clinical Examination

The obstructive airway disorders include asthma, COPD (chronic bronchitis & emphysema) and bronchiectasis. A quick bedside test for obstruction is the 6 second test. If at the beginning of the examination, one asks the patient to take a deep breath in and breath out as fast as they can and if the patient is still expiring after six seconds, an obstructive disease can be suspected. Look for bedside clues like inhalers and home NIV machines.

Classical Signs	Additional Signs
• Tar staining • Prolonged expiratory time • Reduced air entry • Bilateral polyphonic wheeze	• Central cyanosis • Asterixis • Clubbing • Scars • Inhalers

Sample Presentation

This patient has features of airway obstruction as evidenced by prolonged expiratory time, bilateral polyphonic wheeze with reduced air entry throughout the chest. The likely aetiology is cigarette smoking as suggested by the patient's tar stained fingers. There is evidence of central cyanosis and pulmonary hypertension as demonstrated by a loud P2 and a right ventricular heave. There is no clubbing, cyanosis, raised JVP, dependent oedema, lymphadenopathy or asterixis.

There are no features of cor pulmonale. The main differential diagnosis is alpha 1 antitrypsin deficiency.

I would proceed to take a history.

Common discussion topics: Differentials, Investigations & Management.

Differentials: Smoking (main differential); consider Alpha 1 antitrypsin deficiency in young patients.

Investigations	Management
• CXR — hyperinflation (low flat diaphragm, hyper translucent lung fields, tubular heart shadow and the 8th posterior rib is visible above the diaphragm) • ECG — p pulmonale, RV strain • Spirometry — FEV1/FVC <70 % (obstructive picture) • ABG — to assess for respiratory failure.	• Smoking cessation • Inhaled bronchodilators • Steroids ± antibiotics for exacerbations • Non-invasive ventilation for Type 2 respiratory failure • Pulmonary rehabilitation • Lung volume reduction surgery • LTOT (indications are: PO_2 <7.3 or PO_2 < 8 with evidence of cor pulmonale, right heart failure or polycythaemia)

STATION 3A: CARDIOLOGY

Introduction to Cardiology

An important topic we shall cover in this introduction is why candidates fail in the cardiovascular station. A lot of this holds true for other stations as well. The commonest and easiest case in station 3 is that of prosthetic heart valves. Usually the candidate's task is to examine the patient and provide a list of differential diagnoses for the patient's symptoms (commonly dyspnoea or chest pain). The examinee must not get *'taken in'* by the fact that this is the cardiology station and mention both cardiac and non-cardiac causes for symptoms. There are a finite number of cases in this station, but candidates routinely fail the exam in this station due to a few common mistakes.

Before we proceed with this section, we would like to warn the examinee about the easiest failing point in the exam in the cardiology station — the **JVP**. Examinees are expected to decide if there are signs of heart failure (RHF — raised JVP, dependent oedema, enlarged tender liver; LHF — bibasal crackles, gallop rhythm, pulsus alternans), most importantly if the JVP is elevated or not.

The best advice we can give you with regards to not just this case, but the entire cardiology section is this: **DO NOT COMMENT ON A JVP AS RAISED UNLESS YOU ARE ABSOLUTELY SURE AND THERE ARE SUPPORTING EVIDENCE OF RIGHT HEART FAILURE (dependent oedema, enlarged tender liver) and/or PULMONARY HYPERTENSION (loud sounding or palpable P2, left parasternal heave, and/or functional TRICUSPID REGURTITAITON)**. With tricuspid regurgitation, the JVP will be elevated to the angle of the mandible with giant v waves and associated with a left parasternal heave and a holosystolic murmur loudest on inspiration in the left sternal edge. The exceptional case is that of cannon waves in complete heart block where the jugular pulsation will be irregular.

If there are multiple prosthetic valves, *listening without the stethoscope is vital. Bring your ear close to the patient's chest with the left hand on the carotid pulse timing the metallic click*. The metallic click from the mitral valve prosthesis will be loudest over the apex and correspond to S1 (*just preceding the carotid pulsation*) whilst the aortic valve prosthetic click will be loudest over the aortic area and correspond to S2 (*after the carotid pulsation*). Tricuspid valve prosthesis would be loudest over the left sternal edge and the metallic click from their closure would precede the carotid pulsation (i.e. correspond to S1). Mechanical valves are not usually implanted for pulmonary valve disease.

When presenting cases, **DO NOT RUSH to tell the examiner about the murmur** you heard, as a second- or third-year medical student might. The most important part of auscultating the heart is the heart sounds. If the S1 is abnormal, the mitral or tricuspid valves are pathological. On the other hand, an abnormal S2 is a clue towards aortic or pulmonary valve pathology. Then listen for added sounds (S3/S4) and murmurs. **Train your ears to listen for the heart sounds first and then listen for murmurs and time them with a central (NOT PERIPHERAL) pulse.**

The other case candidates find challenging is mixed valve diseases. We shall go on to teach you that with these cases, you must make up your mind which the predominant lesion is. In these cases, the nature of the pulse, apex beat, and the intensity of the heart sounds will guide you towards the culprit lesion. Practise drawing heart sounds you listen to during ward rounds. This helps you visualise the events in each area of the heart whilst you are listening and will help you develop an organised system for listening to heart sounds.

With practice, you should be able to determine the culprit lesion from clues such as the pulse, JVP and general appearance of the patient even before you have placed your stethoscope on the patient's chest. Once you put the stethoscope on the patient's chest listen for S1, S2 then S3, S4 and then listen for murmurs. This entire process should take 4–4.5 minutes with practice and you can then use the extra minute to look for the cause & complications. During presentation describe:

The Pulse — Rate/Rhythm/Volume/Character

Apex Beat — Character and position?

Auscultatory findings — Heart sounds? Added sounds or murmurs? Were the murmurs systolic or diastolic? What part of systole or diastole did you best hear them?

Signs of heart failure or infective endocarditis?

Any peripheral clues as to the cause of the cardiac lesion? E.g. Connective tissue disorders, Psoriasis, Malar flush.

Case 1: Prosthetic Heart Valves

Clinical Examination: The two most important signs to differentiate between metal valves and bio-prosthetic valves.

Classical Signs	Additional Signs
<ul><li>Midline sternotomy scar</li><li>Audible prosthetic valve 'clicks'</li><li>MVR: Metallic S1, Normal S2</li><li>AVR: Normal S1, Metallic S2</li></ul>	<ul><li>Ejection systolic murmur — does not indicate aortic valve dysfunction</li><li>**Diastolic** murmur/collapsing pulse — indicate a dysfunctional metallic aortic valve</li><li>A pansystolic murmur at the apex that **RADIATES** into the left axilla indicates a leaking mitral valve</li><li>Stigmata of infective endocarditis</li><li>Bioprosthetic valves produce no audible clicks but they can produce crisp heart sounds.</li><li>Look for evidence of heart failure (failing valve)</li></ul>

Sample presentation 1: On cardiovascular examination, the patient is comfortable at rest. There is a midline sternotomy scar with an audible prosthetic valve click. The pulse is regular at 60/minute. The blood pressure is ... mmHg. There are no clinical signs of anaemia. The venous pressure is not elevated. The apex beat is palpable in the left 5th intercostal space and normal in character. There are no palpable thrills/heaves. There is a metallic click at the first heart sound followed by a systolic flow murmur loudest over the mitral area with no radiation. The second heart sound is normal and audible in all areas. There are no added sounds. There are no signs of heart failure or infective endocarditis. These features are consistent with a functional metallic mitral valve prosthesis.

Sample presentation 2: On cardiovascular examination, the patient is comfortable at rest. There is a midline sternotomy scar and an audible prosthetic click. The pulse is regular at 80/minute. The blood pressure is ... mmHg. There are no clinical signs of anaemia. The venous pressure is not elevated. The apex beat is palpable in the left 5th intercostal space and normal in character. There are no palpable thrills/heaves. The first heart sound is normal and audible in all areas. There is a crisp second heart sound followed by a systolic flow murmur loudest over the aortic area with no radiation. There are no added sounds or diastolic murmurs. There are no signs of heart failure or infective endocarditis. These features are consistent with a functional metallic aortic valve prosthesis.

Common discussion topics:

- Indications for valve replacement
- What types of valve replacements are there?
- How would a patient with a prosthetic valve be followed up?
- Complications of prosthetic valves.

Choice of mechanical vs. bioprosthetic valve:

Mechanical valves	Bioprosthetic valves
• Patient's desire (no contraindications to long term anticoagulation). • Risk of accelerated structural valve disease. • Already on anticoagulation for a mechanical prosthesis at another site. • < 60 years for AV and < 65 years for MV. • Where redo valve surgery might be risky in a patient with reasonable life expectancy • Patient already on long term anticoagulation due to risk of VTE.	• Patient's desire. • Good quality anticoagulation is unlikely (e.g. Compliance issues; not readily available) or high risk of bleeding (e.g. previous major haemorrhage, comorbidities; unwillingness; compliance issues; lifestyle; occupation). • Re-operation of mechanical valve thrombosis despite good long-term anticoagulant control. • Future re-do surgery low risk. • Young women contemplating pregnancy (weak indication). • Patients > 65 years for AVR and > 70 years for MVR or in patients with life expectancy lower than presumed durability of bio prosthesis.

Note: In patients aged 60–65 years for AVR and 65–70 years for MVR, either type of prosthesis may be used depending on individual characteristics other than age.

Complications of prosthetic valves: FAITH
Failure — valve dehiscence; wear & tear of bioprosthetic valve. **A**rrhythmias, especially AF with MVR. **I**nfective endocarditis **T**hromboembolic phenomena **H**aemorrhage (from anticoagulation) and valve related Haemolysis

Case 2: Aortic Stenosis

Clinical Signs:

Classical signs	Signs of severity
• Low volume, slow rising pulse • Narrow pulse pressure • Heaving apex beat (LVH) • Thrill over aortic area • Ejection click before murmur (indicates pliable valve e.g. bicuspid aortic valve in younger patients) • Soft S2 (this is a sign of severity but it also the most important sign; severe aortic stenosis is unlikely with normal S2) • Ejection systolic murmur (ESM) radiating to the carotids	• Soft and delayed S2 • Prolonged ESM • Audible S4 (also a sign of left heart failure) • Signs of heart failure • Right heart — raised JVP, dependant oedema, enlarged tender liver. • Left heart — pulsus alternans, bibasal crackles, gallop rhythm. • Slow rising pulse • Narrow pulse pressure • Reversed splitting of second heart sound

Presentation:

I examined the cardiovascular system of this 68-year old gentleman who was comfortable at rest. He has a low volume, slow rising pulse at ... beats/minute. The pulse pressure is narrow (.../... mmHg). There are no signs of connective tissue disease. On examination of the precordium, there was a palpable thrill in the aortic area. The second heart sound was soft and associated with an ejection systolic murmur radiating to the carotids best heard loudest with the breath held on expiration. There were no signs of heart failure or infective endocarditis. These features are consistent with a diagnosis of aortic stenosis which I feel is severe based on the presence of a soft S2 and a palpable thrill. I would proceed to take a **full history** for to establish the symptomatic status including angina, syncope and dyspnoea and arrange a transthoracic echocardiogram to confirm my diagnosis and grade severity of aortic stenosis.

Investigations	Management
ECG — voltage criteria for left ventricular hypertrophy (R in V5/6 larger than 25 mm or S in V1 + R in V6 larger than 35 mm) and evidence of AV conduction defects (1/2/3 HB)	**MDT approach,** lifestyle changes, cardiac rehab, treatment of atherosclerosis risk factors. If **symptomatic (Angina, Syncope, Dyspnoea)** → **AVR.**
CXR — calcified valve; cardiomegaly; pulmonary oedema	If AVR contraindicated and long-life expectancy → **TAVI** (transcatheter aortic valve implantation).
Echocardiography — to confirm diagnosis and grade severity by measuring valve area (< 1 cm^2 — severe) and gradient across valve (>40 mm Hg — severe); LV systolic function (if < 50 % — consider surgery).	If AVR contraindicated & short life expectancy → **Medical management** (Digoxin, Diuretics and careful administration of ACEI/ARBs). **Asymptomatic patients:**
Exercise tolerance test — asymptomatic patients with EF >50 % if physically fit	— Other cardiac surgery → AVR — If valve area < 1 cm^2/gradient > 40 mmHg &/or LVEF < 50 % → AVR/TAVI — If LVEF > 50 % & physically active, consider **ETT** → symptomatic/↓BP → consider surgery.
Coronary angiogram — rule out coronary artery disease; discuss in cardiothoracic MDT for CABG +/-AVR.	

Other differential diagnoses of an ejection systolic murmur:

- Aortic sclerosis (murmur does not radiate to carotids)
- Aortic flow murmur (high output states — anaemia, pregnancy and hyperthyroidism)
- Hypertrophic obstructive cardiomyopathy (jerky pulse; double apical impulse; normal S2; louder on crouching)

Mention the other differentials of a systolic murmur (MR, TR, and VSD) ONLY if the murmur does not radiate to the carotids.

Aetiology of aortic stenosis:
- Age related degeneration (calcified aortic valve)
- Bicuspid aortic valve (congenital)
- Rheumatic valvular heart disease
- William's syndrome (supravalvular aortic stenosis)

Case 3: Aortic Regurgitation

Clinical Examination:

Classical signs	Additional signs
• Large volume, collapsing pulse • Wide pulse pressure • Head nodding (de Musset's sign) • Visible carotid pulsations (Corrigan's sign) • Capillary pulsation in the fingernails (Quincke's sign) • Pistol shot femoral pulse (Traube's sign) • Displaced, thrusting apex beat • Early diastolic high-pitched murmur best heard in the left sternal edge with the patient sitting forward breath held on expiration.	Stigmata of connective tissue disorders (Marfan's syndrome, ankylosing spondylitis, rheumatoid arthritis) Other murmurs – • Austin Flint murmur (mid diastolic rumble due to turbulent mixing of retrograde AR and anterograde Mitral valve flow within the LV). • Systolic flow murmur
Signs of severity	
• Wide pulse pressure • Collapsing pulse • Prolonged duration of early diastolic murmur • Signs of heart failure • Presence of Austin Flint murmur	

Presentation: The patient is comfortable at rest. He has a large volume, collapsing rising pulse with wide pulse pressure .../... mmHg). On examination of the precordium, there was a palpable thrill in the aortic area/left sternal edge. The apex beat was displaced to the left consistent with volume overload. The second heart sound was soft and associated with a diastolic murmur best heard in the aortic area/left sternal edge with the patient sitting forward breath held on expiration. There was evidence of hyperdynamic circulation as evidenced by Corrigan's sign, De Musset's sign, Quincke's sign and Duroziez's sign. The patient is clinically euvolaemic and has no signs of heart failure or stigmata of infective endocarditis. These features are consistent with a diagnosis of aortic regurgitation likely secondary to…. (MENTION YOUR DIFFERENTIAL DIAGNOSIS). I would like to take a fully history to establish the patient's symptomatic status and arrange a transthoracic echocardiogram to confirm my diagnosis and rule out other aortic pathology.

Aetiology of aortic incompetence: Common causes in bold

	Acute	Chronic
Valve leaflet	• **Infective endocarditis** • **Prosthetic valve paravalvular leakage/failure** • Ruptured sinus of Valsalva • Acute rheumatic fever (rare in the West)	• **Bicuspid aortic valve** • **Rheumatic valvular heart disease**
Aortic Root	• Aortic dissection (Type A) • Trauma	Aortic root dilatation — • **Marfan's syndrome** • **Hypertension** • Aorto-annular ectasia Aortitis – • Connective tissue disorders (**Ankylosing spondylitis**, Psoriatic arthritis, Osteogenesis imperfecta) • **Treponemal disease**

	Aortic stenosis	Aortic regurgitation
Pulse	Slow rising	Collapsing
Pulse pressure	Narrow	Wide
Apex beat	Heaving, pressure loaded, not displaced	Thrusting, volume loaded, displaced
Heart sounds	Soft S2; normal S1	Soft S2, S1 usually normal unless there is an Austin flint murmur
Murmur	ESM	EDM

MIXED AORTIC VALVULAR DISEASE: Try to identify the predominant lesion from the apex beat and pulse. Management is guided by treatment of the predominant valvular lesion as discussed in cardiothoracic MDTs based on individual patient's symptomatic status and echocardiographic findings. Especially in younger patients with congenital valve problems, there now is a trend towards offering aortic valve repair. Symptoms (for pressure overload) and decompensated LV function (for volume overload) are indications for surgery.

Case 4: Mitral Stenosis

Clinical Examination:

Classical signs	Additional signs
<ul><li>Malar flush</li><li>Irregular pulse</li><li>Tapping apex beat</li><li>Opening snap</li><li>Loud S1</li><li>Low pitched localised RuMBLe[2]</li></ul>	<ul><li>Signs of infective endocarditis</li><li>Left thoracotomy scar (previous mitral valvotomy)</li></ul>

Sample Presentation:

I examined the cardiovascular system of this 45-year-old lady who was comfortable at rest. There was a visible malar flush. The pulse rate was 60/min, irregular and small volume. The apex beat was palpable in the left fifth intercostal space in the mid clavicular line and tapping in character. The first heart sound is clearly audible and loud and (maybe) associated with an opening snap. The second heart sound was normal. There was a Low pitched Localised Rough Rumbling Mid diastolic Murmur loudest in the apical area best heard with the Bell of the stethoscope with the patient in Left Lateral position and with the breath held on expiration. (MNEMONIC: LLRRMMBBLL — Low pitched Localized RuMBLe[2]). There are no signs/signs of pulmonary hypertension and heart failure or stigmata of infective endocarditis. These features are consistent with mitral stenosis. I would like to take a full history to establish the symptomatic status and any past medical history rheumatic valvular heart disease. Any history of weight loss or lethargy could be in keeping with a differential diagnosis of atrial myxoma (TUMOUR PLOP). In presence of pulmonary hypertension, the P2 component of S2 may be loud and palpable with associated left parasternal heave. Presystolic accentuation of the murmur is absent if the patient is in AF.

Differential diagnosis of mid diastolic murmur	Aetiology of mitral stenosis
<ul><li>Mitral stenosis</li><li>Left atrial myxoma (Tumour plop)</li><li>Austin Flint murmur (See case: Aortic incompetence)</li><li>Ball valve thrombus in left atrium.</li></ul>	<ul><li>Rheumatic valvular heart disease (RVHD)</li><li>Calcification of valve (degenerative)</li><li>Endocarditis</li><li>Carcinoid syndrome</li><li>Congenital (cleft valve) (rare)</li></ul>
Investigations	Management
<ul><li>**ECG** — AF, p mitrale</li><li>**CXR** — enlarged left atrium (splaying of carina), pulmonary oedema, calcification</li><li>**Transthoracic Echocardiogram** to confirm diagnosis, assess the severity and consequences of MS, as well as the extent of anatomic lesions. MS does not usually have clinical consequences at rest when valve area is 1.5 cm^2. Echocardiography also evaluates pulmonary artery pressures, associated MR, concomitant valve disease, and LA size.</li><li>**Transoesophageal echocardiography (TOE)** helps exclude LA thrombus before PMC (per cutaneous mitral commissurotomy) or after an embolic episode.</li></ul>	Options include:<ul><li>**General supportive measures**: Multidisciplinary approach, early specialist intervention, patient education, smoking cessation</li><li>**Medical management**: Treatment of heart failure and Treatment of AF (rate control/rhythm control/anticoagulation) as per ESC guidelines.</li><li>**Primary mitral commissurotomy (PMC)** — balloon valvotomy (procedure of choice)</li><li>**Surgery** — closed mitral valvotomy, open valvotomy (now rarely done), valve replacement.</li></ul>

Case 5: Pansystolic Murmurs

5A — Mitral Incompetence

Clinical Examination:

Classical signs	Additional signs
• Irregularly irregular pulse (if patient in AF). • Displaced, thrusting apex. • Systolic thrill. • Soft S1. • PSM loudest in the mitral area best heard in the left lateral position with the breath held on expiration. • Radiation of murmur to axilla. • S3 — due to rapid ventricular filling (giving a gallop rhythm; this virtually rules out MS). • Wide splitting of S2 (with severe MR due to early closure of aortic valve due to low presystolic LV volume). • S4 (in sinus rhythm)	• Signs of heart failure: LHF — bibasal crackles, gallop rhythm, pulsus alternans. RHF — raised JVP, dependent oedema, enlarged tender liver. • Signs of pulmonary hypertension/RV hypertrophy — Raised JVP with CV waves suggestive of severe functional TR, palpable P2, left parasternal heave, dependent oedema. • MS + MR — added MDM — NO ROLE OF VALVE REPAIR. • Features of infective endocarditis • Stigmata of connective tissue disorder

Sample Presentation: On cardiovascular examination, the patient is comfortable at rest. The pulse rate was 60/minute and irregular & small volume *(if in AF)*. On examination of the precordium, the apex beat was thrusting in nature and displaced to the anterior axillary line in the left 6th intercostal space. There was an apical thrill. On auscultation, the first heart was soft, but the second heart sound was clearly audible and normal in character *(With severe MR, there may be a wide split S2 and/ or an S3 due to rapid ventricular filling)*. There was a pansystolic murmur loudest in the apical area radiating towards the left axilla best heard in left lateral position with the breath held on expiration. The venous pressure is elevated and there is evidence of ankle or sacral oedema *(If there are no features of volume overload, mention that the patient is euvolaemic and has no signs of heart failure. Beware the patient who is euvolaemic — If you don't do all the manoeuvres you might not hear the murmur at all & hear only a very soft S1)*. There are no peripheral stigmata of infective endocarditis. These features are consistent with a diagnosis of severe mitral regurgitation complicated by cardiac failure.

Then mention that the chief differential diagnosis of a pansystolic murmur are tricuspid regurgitation (best heard in the left parasternal area on inspiration; NOTE — a functional TR is expected with severe MR) and ventricular septal defect (usually young patient; once again in the left parasternal area with no change with respiration. Mention that in presence of a soft S1 a VSD is highly unlikely).

The top causes are **infective endocarditis, rheumatic valvular heart disease, age related degeneration (calcification), ischaemic heart disease and MV prolapse.**

Congenital Causes	Acquired Causes
• **Mitral valve prolapse:** Associated with ASD secundum; Polycystic kidney disease & Turner's syndrome (look for the signs in a short statured female)	• **Rheumatic valvular heart disease** • **Infective endocarditis** • **Calcification** • Connective tissue disorders • Functional MR (secondary to dilated LV due to any cause — cardiomyopathies — ischaemic/drug induced esp. chemotherapy/congenital cardiomyopathies) • **Ischaemic heart disease:** Papillary muscle rupture (usually after an MI); Ischaemic cardiomyopathy causing LV dilatation
Investigations	
• ECG: AF, p Mitrale • CXR: pulmonary congestion, cardiomegaly, enlarge LA • TTE/TOE: To confirm diagnosis, assess severity (including size of MR jet, LV dimensions and EF)	
Management	

Acute severe mitral incompetence (e.g. Infective endocarditis, ruptured chordae tendineae) → emergency surgery might be indicated.

For chronic mitral incompetence, the indications of **surgery** are as follows.

Symptomatic patients:

1. LVEF > 30 %.
2. LVEF < 30 % refractory to medical therapy where durable valve repair is likely, and morbidity is low.

Asymptomatic patients:

1. LVEF < 60 % or LVESD (left ventricular end systolic diameter) > 45 mm.
2. New onset AF or Systolic Pulmonary artery pressure (SPAP) > 50 mmHg.

Medical management is indicated in symptomatic patients with LVEF < 30 %. If these patients are refractory to medical management surgery may be concerned only if durable valve repair is likely with low morbidity.

Medical management also involves follow-up with annual echocardiography and treatment of heart failure and AF (rate control/ rhythm control/ anticoagulation) as per ESC guidelines.

NOTE ON MIXED MITRAL VALVE DISEASE

Try to identify the predominant lesion from the location and nature of the apex beat (undisplaced tapping apex — MS; displaced heaving apex — MR). As with mixed aortic valve disease, the key aspect of assessment is the candidate's ability to determine the dominant lesion. Investigations include 12 lead ECG, Chest X ray and Echocardiography. Please note that in patients with severe pulmonary hypertension, either isolated or in association with mitral stenosis, there is usually associated functional tricuspid regurgitation, the pan-systolic murmur of which can mimic mitral regurgitation. In this situation, remember that tricuspid regurgitation is associated with giant v waves and a pansystolic murmur that is louder in inspiration and will be loudest over the lower left sternal edge. The liver will be pulsatile. The murmur of mitral incompetence is louder in expiration and radiates to the left axilla.

Management: Although treatment depends on the predominant lesion, there is **no role of per cutaneous valvuloplasty** in mixed mitral valve disease. The treatment options are medical management or surgical valve replacement based on symptoms and/or echocardiographic features.

5B — Tricuspid Regurgitation

Clinical Examination:

Classical signs	Additional signs

• Raised JVP with prominent 'v' waves.
• Quiet S1
• Loud P2
• PSM over lower left sternal edge, loudest on inspiration
• Remember:
  o **RI**-ght- **Right** sided murmurs heard louder in **Inspiration**
  o **LE**-ft — **Left** sided murmurs heard louder in **Expiration**
	• Signs of right heart failure — pulsatile hepatomegaly, dependent oedema.
	• Clues about aetiology — multiple needle marks (IVDU); hyperexpanded chest, cyanosis, polyphonic wheeze (COPD); other signs of respiratory disease.

Causes of TR
• Functional (secondary to dilated annulus) • Secondary to pulmonary hypertension (cor pulmonale, CCF) • RVHD • Infective endocarditis (esp. IVDU) • Carcinoid syndrome • Ebstein's anomaly (atrialisation of right ventricle)

Investigations	Management
• ECG: RVH, p Pulmonale • CXR: enlarged RA (double right heart border • TTE/TOE: diagnosis and severity; RV dimensions.	• Tricuspid annuloplasty or valve replacement.

Indications of tricuspid valve surgery:

Tricuspid stenosis: Symptomatic severe TS or patient undergoing left sided heart intervention.

Tricuspid Regurgitation:

Absolute indications	Relative indications
• Symptomatic patients with severe isolated primary TR without severe right ventricular dysfunction. • Severe primary or secondary TR in patients undergoing left sided valve surgery.	• Moderate primary TR undergoing left sided valve surgery. • Mild — moderate secondary TR with dilated annulus (≥ 40 mm or ≥ 21 mm/m^2). • Asymptomatic patients with severe isolated TR with progressively worsening RV function/RV dilatation. • Symptomatic patients with severe TR after left sided heart surgery with progressive RV dilatation/dysfunction (in absence of left heart valve dysfunction, severe RV/LV Dysfunction, and severe pulmonary vascular disease).

5C — Ventricular Septal Defects

Clinical Examination:

Classical signs	Additional signs
<ul><li>Usually a young patient.</li><li>Undisplaced apex.</li><li>Thrill at left sternal edge.</li><li>Harsh pansystolic murmur at left sternal edge that DOES NOT RADIATE OR CHANGE WITH RESPIRATION. Usually heart sounds are normal in haemodynamically non-significant VSDs.</li></ul>	<ul><li>The apex beat may be displaced with a haemodynamically significant VSD (volume overload).</li><li>With the development of Eisenmenger's or shunt reversal, the murmur becomes quiet and a functional TR might develop with worsening pulmonary hypertension. The murmur will become louder on inspiration (Carvallo's sign) with development of signs of CCF. Only a single loud S2 is audible and there might be development of clubbing and cyanosis. It would be clinically impossible to differentiate from a TR without echocardiography.</li><li>In large VSDs, due to increased preload and flow through the mitral valve, a mid-diastolic apical rumble becomes audible.</li></ul>
Types	**Complications**
<ul><li>Perimembranous (80%)</li><li>Infundibular (5–8%)</li><li>Muscular (5–20 %)</li><li>Posterior (8–10 %).</li></ul>	<ul><li>Pulmonary hypertension</li><li>LVF</li><li>Endocarditis</li><li>AR</li><li>Arrhythmias (esp. VT, VF)</li><li>Eisenmenger's syndrome.</li></ul>
**Causes**	
<ul><li>Congenital — Aneuploidies (Down's, Edwards, Patau's, Di George)</li><li>Acquired — IHD (Post MI septal rupture); Iatrogenic (RV pacing; complication of septal ablation procedures)</li></ul>	

Investigations	Management
• ECG: Bundle branch block, LVH (volume overload), Katz Wachtel phenomenon (voltage > 50 mm in V2 — V4 due to biventricular hypertrophy), p mitrale (Left atrial hypertrophy) • CXR: oligaemic lung fields, cardiomegaly, LA hypertrophy (double right heart border) • TTE/TOE: diagnosis (best in subcostal views), size & direction of shunt, ventricular dimensions & function • Qp:Qs ratio > 2:1 (pulmonary: systemic flow) is an indication for surgery. • Catheterisation as part of workup for closure	• Clinically non-significant VSDs with normal PA pressures do not need surgery and often close spontaneously (except infundibular defects). • However, haemodynamically significant VSDs may be considered for percutaneous device or surgical closure prior to development of Eisenmenger syndrome. Contra-indicated in presence of severe pulmonary hypertension.

Indications for surgery
• Acute septal rupture • Symptomatic patients with no severe pulmonary vascular disease. • Qp:Qs ratio > 2:1 (pulmonary: systemic flow) • Volume overload (even if asymptomatic) • Recurrent endocarditis. • Progressive aortic incompetence (VSD associated AV cusp prolapse) • VSD + Pulmonary arterial hypertension (PAH) — can be considered for surgery while there is still net L-R shunt (Pulmonary: Systemic flow ratio aka Qp: Qs > 1.5) and pulmonary arterial pressure (PAP) or pulmonary arterial hypertension (PAH) are < 2/3 systemic values. This can be at baseline or after NO challenge, or after targeted treatment of PAH.

STATION 3B: NEUROLOGY

Introduction to the Neurology Section

Candidates are often unnecessarily stressed by this station. As far as the general medicine trainee's ability to quantify neurological disease, one is not always expected to make a definitive diagnosis in the PACES exam. However, a systematic approach is expected when examining patients. In this introductory section, we shall attempt to provide some brief guidelines.

The commonest instructions in the examination are as follows.

- Examine the patient neurologically (there is a multisystem disease or disease involving both upper and lower limb e.g. Parkinson's or cerebellar syndrome) — the easiest trick is to start with gait and speech in these stations.
- Examine the speech. Unfortunately, there are few books which provide a simple system to do this simultaneously addressing pathology. A section on this will follow.
- Examine the cranial nerves and proceed accordingly. Think of the cranial nerves in being affected in groups. Often, the examiners expect you to pick up pathology not directly affecting the cranial nerves such as demyelination (relative afferent pupillary defect), cerebellar syndrome (nystagmus, dysarthria) or specific facies (myotonic facies). Therefore, practise doing the entire cranial nerve examination in 3 minutes to give you time to exhibit signs of other disease.
- Examine the upper/lower limbs neurologically.

Proceed systematically guided by the following sections — 'The Two Weeks to PACES' (2W2P) methods for neurological examination of limbs & speech. Before starting, greet the patient and always remember to seek permission to expose the patient and offer to cover the patient afterwards. Neurology is all about giving the right instructions. Learn from an expert and memorise the instructions you are going to give for every step. Do not be over concerned about specific deficits or weakness in a movement. Concentrate on whether the deficit is proximal or distal, flexor or extensor, sensory, motor or sensorimotor, unilateral or bilateral. Decide if this is an upper or a lower motor neuron lesion and if there is a specific sensory level.

Neurological Examination of Limbs — 2W2P Method

Inspection	Screening Manoeuvres	Examination Proper
• Look at the patient as a whole. Is there an obvious diagnosis? • Pay close attention to age, sex ethnicity, posture, face, hands, feet. • Are the examiners trying to hide an obvious clue (e.g. asking you to examine upper limbs leaving lower limbs covered) • Bedside clues (Catheters, Shoes/Walking aids/ Wheelchairs) • Is there an ophthalmoscope? • Any obvious tremors? Then check DWARFS: • **Deformities** • **Wasting** • **Asymmetry** • **Redness** • **Fasciculation** (lower motor neuron pathology). • **Scars: ALWAYS EXAMINE THE SPINE FIRST.**	Upper limbs: • Pronator Drift (UMN disease) • Myotonia (patient to grip your hands or make a fist & release) • Bradykinesia (slow & reduced amplitude when patient asked to repeatedly bring thumb & forefinger together). • Rebound phenomenon (cerebellar dysfunction) • Fatiguability by counting from 1 – 30 (Myasthenia) if you find ptosis and patient looks lethargic. Lower limbs: • Romberg's test. • Gait (Ask permission to walk the patient).	• Tone • Power • Reflexes • Coordination • Sensation If previous examination showed LMN signs, check gloves & stockings first. Otherwise check for a sensory level first. **If you were not allowed to examine gait first by the examiner, don't forget to check this or mention it at the end if you run out of time.** Ask yourself the following questions about the lesion or neurological deficit as you examine. • Proximal/distal? • Flexor/extensor? • Sensory, motor or sensorimotor? • Unilateral/Bilateral? • UMNL, LMNL, a neuro-muscular junction problem or a pure myopathy? • Is there a sensory level?

Be familiar with the 8 basic pathological gaits.

- Hemiplegic
- Spastic diplegic
- Neuropathic
- Myopathic
- Parkinsonian
- Choreiform
- Ataxic
- Sensory

NEVER WALK AWAY FROM ANY NEUROLOGICAL EXAMINATION WITHOUT EXAMINING THE SPINE. To complete the examination, mention that you would like to examine the set of limbs you haven't examined and the cranial nerves. You would then proceed to take a full history including onset, duration, progression, aggravating & relieving factors as well as associated features including past medical history, personal history, family history and drug history.

Then proceed to present your findings in the exact order you examined (INSPECTION, SCREENING TESTS if positive, TONE, POWER, REFELXES, COORDINATION, SENSATION). The above method allows you to pick up or rule out certain common PACES cases early.

When asked about management of neurological disease, the answer should always begin as follows, *"I would like to manage this patient in a multidisciplinary approach with early involvement of specialist physicians, physiotherapy, occupational therapy and neurological rehabilitation services with focus on patient & family education. Specific management will depend on the cause."* Memorise this line prior to the exam.

The presentation should highlight the following (5 Cs).

- **C**ondition
- **C**ause
- **C**omplications (of disease & treatment)
- Effect of patient's functional **C**apacity
- Need to address patient's & carers' **C**oncerns.

The 2W2P modified surgical sieve for neurology is a 'Get out of jail free' card when queried about differential diagnoses, especially with *upper motor neuron or cerebellar pathology*. It also helps formulate a thought process for the non-specialist physician to use when thinking about neurological illness.

Neurological illness can be classified as follows.

A. Congenital
B. Acquired:

- TrAuMA = **Tr**auma, **Au**toimmune, **M**etabolic (including diabetes, **A**lcohol (& drugs)
- Tumour
- Infection
- Infarction (i.e. Vascular)
- Demyelination

Common conditions must be mentioned first when asked about differential diagnoses. Be guided by examination findings when presenting differentials.

Examining Speech — The 2W2P Method

It is important to have a clear idea about speech and language problems as one proceeds to the speech examination. This station is often a source of worry for most candidates mainly because it is taught poorly and practised infrequently.

We shall provide a method but the only way to be proficient at it is to practise this method at least once a day leading up to the examination. You do not need a patient to practise this. It can be completed in 3 minutes leaving you time to proceed with further examination to demonstrate additional signs if indicated. Remember you are assessing articulation, phonation and speech reception, comprehension & expression.

Dysarthria	Dysphonia	Dysphasia
• Pseudobulbar palsy (spastic dysarthria — UMNL IX, X & XII) • Bulbar palsy (LMNL IX, X & XII) • Extrapyramidal (low pitched monotonous) • Cerebellar (scanning staccato speech) • Fatigue • Local lesions (tongue, lip, mouth)	• Vocal cord pathology. • Damage to recurrent laryngeal nerve (Tenth n. palsy)	• Expressive (Broca's area) • Receptive (Wernicke's area) • Conductive (Arcuate Fasciculus — check repetition) • Global (all the above) • Dominant parietal lobe (Dyscalculia, Dysgraphia, Dyslexia).

The TWO WEEKS TO PACES 10 step speech examination:

1. Spontaneous speech: Ask the patient his name & how he got to the hospital.
   Assess volume & tone (extrapyramidal dysarthria), clarity (dysarthria, dysphonia) & fluency (global dysphasia). Look for neologisms & paraphasias (sensory dysphasia); reduced number of words & telegraphic speech (expressive dysphasia).
2. Ask the patient to say, 'Yellow Lorry, Hello Lorry' (checking for bulbar palsy as in this lower motor neuron lesion, nasal & lingual sounds are altered).
3. Ask the patient to say, 'Baby hippopotamus' (this simultaneously assesses consonants altered in pseudobulbar palsy & for cerebellar dysarthria).
4. Ask the patient to say, 'West Register Street' (cerebellar dysarthria).
5. Ask patient to count to thirty (checking for fatiguability).

6. Ask patient to cough and then say 'Aaah' (vocal cord function; dysphonia). Look at the tongue and uvula. Is there any evidence of bulbar/pseudobulbar palsy? Offer to check jaw jerk (pseudobulbar palsy).
7. Ask patient to name a common object (e.g. pen/watch) (Nominal dysphasia).
8. Ask patient to follow a three-stage command (e.g. Pick up this sheet of paper, fold it in half and put it back) to check for sensory dysphasia. Go and stand behind the patient to ensure you are not giving visual clues.
9. Ask patient to repeat 'Today is Tuesday' (checking for conductive dysphasia).
10. Check the function of the dominant parietal lobe.
    DYSLEXIA: 'Could you read the first sentence on this page?'
    DYSGRAPHIA: 'Can you please write a sentence?'
    DYSCALCULIA: Please add 3 + 2.

Case 1: Extrapyramidal Syndrome

Clinical Examination

Classical Signs	Additional Signs
• Expressionless face • Decreased blinking • Monotonous tone of voice • Asymmetrical 'pill-rolling' **tremor** • Lead pipe **rigidity** • Stooped posture and festinating gait with reduced arm swing • **Bradykinesia**: demonstrated by asking patient to walk	• Vertical gaze palsy (Progressive supranuclear palsy) • Autonomic symptoms (Shy-Drager syndrome) • Rarely, cerebellar signs (Multiple system atrophy) • Dementia (Lewy Body) • Apomorphine pumps

Presentation should focus on a) hypokinesis b) phenomenology c) distribution & d) further information needed.

Sample presentation: This elderly gentleman has a mask like expressionless face with monotonous speech. There is evidence of a 3 — 5 Hz pill rolling tremor in his hands associated with asymmetric lead pipe rigidity at the elbows, left more than right. Bradykinesia is demonstrated by reduced amplitude of movements. There is difficulty initiating voluntary movements. The patient walks with a shuffling, narrow based gait & stooped posture with reduced arm swing, left more than right. There is no evidence of up gaze palsy or cerebellar signs.

These features of a kinetic rigidity & tremor are consistent with Parkinsonism & I would like to suggest an aetiology of Idiopathic Parkinson's Disease based on the evidence of asymmetry. Other differentials to be excluded include the Parkinson's plus syndromes, Structural basal ganglia lesions & Drug induced Parkinsonism.

I would like to check for evidence of autonomic dysfunction including postural hypotension, cognitive function and assess handwriting for micrographia. A full history of onset, duration & progression of systems is needed including past medical history, family history & a complete drug history.

Common discussion topics: Pathophysiology of & differentials; Confirmation of diagnosis; treatment strategies and common side effects.

Differential diagnoses (mention causes in bold first)

- **Idiopathic Parkinson's disease**
- **Parkinson's plus syndromes**
  Multisystem atrophy
  Progressive supranuclear palsy
  Corticobasal degeneration; unilateral signs; 60 % have alien hand syndrome
- **Structural lesions in basal ganglia** (trauma, tumour)
- **Drug induced Parkinsonism** (Antipsychotics & other Dopamine depleting medications. e.g. Metoclopramide, Sodium valproate)
- Vascular Parkinsonism (infarction/atherosclerosis)
- Anoxic injury to the basal ganglia (e.g. post-arrest).
- Post encephalitis (encephalitis lethargica)
- Dementia pugilistica (Trauma)
- Toxins (Carbon monoxide, MPTP — a narcotic recreational drug)
- Metabolic causes — Wilson's disease

Investigations	Management
• Diagnosis is predominantly clinical. • *Substantiating criteria for Parkinson's disease include* unilateral signs, symptoms progress over several years, good initial response to Levodopa. • *MRI Brain usually normal* but can be used to rule out structural causes • *DaTscan* can demonstrate reduction in dopamine transporter binding in the early stages.	• Multidisciplinary approach — as mentioned in introduction • Elderly patients are usually started on Levodopa with peripheral DOPA Decarboxylase inhibitors as first line. • Dopamine agonists may be used in mild disease or alongside Levodopa. However, in younger patients these may be used as first line agents to delay the usage of Levodopa. Apomorphine can be used subcutaneously. • COMT inhibitors — may be useful adjunct during any stage of disease • Anticholinergics — useful for tremor • Surgery & Deep brain stimulation techniques have proven benefits.

Case 2: Myotonic Dystrophy

Clinical Examination

Classical Signs	Additional Signs of Complications
• Frontal balding • Bilateral ptosis • Wasting of temporalis, masseters & sternocleidomastoid • Dysarthria • Symmetrical weakness of distal muscles • Myotonic grip (slow release) • Lower motor neuron signs • Percussion myotonia	• Cataracts • Cardiomyopathy — listen for regurgitant murmurs; sigs of heart failure. • AV conduction defects — Pacemakers. • Diabetes mellitus — finger prick marks & insulin injection sites. • Nodular thyroid enlargement ± thyroidectomy scar. • Testicular atrophy & Gynaecomastia (hypogonadism)

Sample Presentation

This patient has features consistent with myotonic dystrophy type 1 as evidenced by a myopathic facies (frontal balding, wasted frontotemporalis) bilateral ptosis and cataracts. Myotonia is evidenced by slow release of grip and difficulty in opening his eyes after firm closure. There is distal wasting & weakness of muscles with depressed deep tendon reflexes and foot drop.

I would like to proceed by dipsticking the urine for glucose, checking BMs for diabetes and listening to the patient's heart for regurgitant murmurs to check for cardiomyopathy. Further investigations will be guided by a full history including family history of respiratory complications following anaesthesia.

Common Discussion topics: Definition, Inheritance, Investigations, Management.

Dystrophia Myotonica = DM = Diabetes Mellitus, Dilated cardio Myopathy

Please note that the above is the classical (Type 1) myotonic dystrophy (autosomal dominant trinucleotide repeat disorder with CTG expansions within the DMPK gene on chromosome 19). Type 2 is a CCTG repeat expansion within ZNF9 gene on chromosome 3 and presents with a similar phenotype but with proximal rather than distal wasting & weakness.

Differential diagnoses: Diagnosis is clinical, but it might a good idea to learn about causes of ptosis, other trinucleotide repeat disorders and causes of myotonia & distal weakness.

Investigations	Management
• Clinical diagnosis • Electromyography ('dive bomber' potentials) • Slit lamp examination for cataracts • OGTT, HbA1c for diabetes • Echocardiography- cardiomyopathy	• No treatment alters course of progressive weakness. • Phenytoin for myotonia • Genetic counselling; warn about **genetic anticipation** • Supportive, multidisciplinary approach • Avoid general anaesthetic • Treatment of complications

Other trinucleotide repeat disorders: Huntington's chorea, Friedrich's ataxia, Spinocerebellar ataxia, Fragile X syndrome.

Unilateral Ptosis	Bilateral Ptosis
• Third nerve palsy • Horner's syndrome	• Myotonic dystrophy • Myasthenia gravis (*Case 5*) • Congenital including mitochondrial myopathies

Case 3: Cerebellar Syndrome

Clinical Examination: Classical Signs

Speech	Eyes
Scanning dysarthria — slurred, staccato speech ('West register street')	Jerky nystagmus (fast phase towards side of lesion)
Upper Limbs (ipsilateral to lesion)	**Lower Limbs (ipsilateral to lesion)**
• Rebound phenomenon • Intention tremor • Dysdiadochokinesis • Dysmetria (past pointing) • Hypotonia • Hyporeflexia	• Heel Shin test +ve • Hypotonia • Hyporeflexia, pendular knee jerks. • 'Broad based' ataxic gait
Additional Signs (suggestive of aetiology)	
• Scars from previous accidents, neurosurgery (post traumatic or SOL) • Cerebellopontine angle syndrome — loss of corneal reflex & sensation (V), facial nerve palsy (VII), unilateral hearing loss (VIII) • Demyelination — Relative afferent pupillary defect; wheelchair bound Caucasian/Northern European; female sex; optic atrophy. • Friedrich's ataxia — absent ankle jerk with extensor planters; dorsal column & pyramidal tract signs; optic atrophy (Please see case 6B) • Phenytoin — gum hypertrophy. • Hypothyroidism — Typical facies; Dry skin; Slow relaxation of reflexes. • Alcoholism — unkempt appearance; peripheral neuropathy; stigmata of chronic liver disease and/or portal hypertension.	

Candidates may be asked to examine cranial nerves, speech, upper or lower limbs or gait. Ensure that you systematically finish the full examination you were originally assigned and then having picked up the neurological deficit in your examination, proceed to exhibit the relevant clinical signs of cerebellar dysfunction in this order: speech, eyes, upper limbs, lower limbs gait and present accordingly. If you run out of time, mention the missing pieces in your presentation. This candidate was asked to examine cranial nerves.

Sample Presentation: The patient is a young, Caucasian female in a wheelchair. Her speech had a slurred, staccato character. Examination of the cranial nerves revealed a jerky nystagmus with the fast phase to the right. There were no other neurological deficits on examination of the cranial nerves. Further examination of upper limbs reveals a positive rebound phenomenon, intention tremor, past pointing, hypotonia & hyporeflexia worse on the right. I would like to complete my examination by performing a full neurological examination of both upper and lower limbs including gait to look for evidence of ataxia and fundoscopy to check for optic atrophy. These features are consistent with a right sided cerebellar lesion and I would like to suggest demyelination as the possible aetiology in view of patient's age, sex & ethnicity. Other differentials include cerebellar trauma, intracranial space occupying lesions (ICSOL) including tumours & abscesses, cerebrovascular events, paraneoplastic syndromes & drugs/toxins including phenytoin and alcohol. A full history of onset, duration, progression and aggravating & relieving factors is needed along with past medical history, drug history, personal history including history of alcohol abuse and a full family history to rule out hereditary causes such as Friedrich's ataxia, Ataxia telangiectasia & Spinocerebellar ataxia.

Common Discussion Topics

- Differential diagnoses,
- Investigations,
- Causes of ataxia & nystagmus.

Differential diagnoses: Use mnemonic PASTRIES in bold or TrAuMA/Tumour/Infection/Infarction/Demyelination).

Acquired	Congenital (Rare)
- Trauma - Tumours & Infections — ICSOL (Intracranial space occupying lesions) - Paraneoplastic syndromes - Infarction (Brainstem Stroke) - Demyelination (**M**S) - Metabolic: B12 deficiency, Hypothyroidism (Endocrine) - Drugs/Toxins: Alcohol, Phenytoin, Lithium (Iatrogenic)	- Hereditary ataxias — Friedrich's ataxia Spinocerebellar ataxias Ataxia telangiectasia

Investigations	Management
- MRI brain (rule out ICSOL) - CSF oligoclonal bands suggest inflammation and are not specific for demyelination. - Vitamin B12 levels. - Thyroid function tests. - Liver function tests. - Phenytoin levels.	- Multidisciplinary approach to maintain independence with ADLs. - Treatment of cause.

Case 4: Peripheral Neuropathy

Clinical Examination

Classical Signs	Signs Related to Aetiology

• Impaired sensation to all modalities
   ✓ Dorsal column (large fibre) — Vibration, Position
   ✓ Spinothalamic tract (small fibres) — Pin prick, Temperature
• 'Gloves & stockings' distribution
• Trophic changes
• Distal LMN type weakness
• Diminished reflexes
• High stepping gait
• Romberg's might be positive
	• Diabetes — Fingerprick marks of blood glucose checks, Lipodystrophy in insulin injection sites, Insulin pens/pumps, diabetic feet with Charcot joints, diabetic dermopathy, proximal myopathy (diabetic amyotrophy), cataracts, offer to do ophthalmoscopy.
	• Charcot Marie Tooth disease — see supplementary case.
	• Uraemia — Signs of renal replacement therapy.
	• Vasculitis — Rashes, Signs of connective tissue disease.
	• Paraneoplastic syndromes — Cancer cachexia, Radiotherapy tattoos.

Sample Presentation: On examination of the lower limbs, I note an insulin pen on the bedside and fingerprick marks from regular BM checks. The lower limbs exhibit trophic changes with shiny & dry skin and hair loss up to the mid shin. I also note evidence of diabetic dermopathy. There is evidence of deformed ankle joints with ulcers and callosities on the heel of the feet. I note the presence of pressure offloading orthotics. The tone is preserved. Proximal myopathy is evidenced by difficulty standing from sitting. Reflexes & coordination were preserved. There is evidence of loss of 'pin prick' sensation up to the mid shin in a stocking distribution as well as loss of dorsal column function (vibration & proprioception). The patient walks with a high stepping gait and Romberg's test is positive. These features are consistent with a diagnosis of peripheral neuropathy and the most likely aetiology is diabetes mellitus. To complete my examination, I would proceed by taking a full history of onset, duration & progression of symptoms, a complete drug history and past medical history and review recent blood glucose records & HbA1c. I would also like to rule out any co-existing autonomic dysfunctions.

Causes: Mention **DIABETES, ALCOHOL, B12 DEFICIENCY & DRUGS** first.

Sensory: (DIABETES...then A, B, C...H, I)

- **Diabetes mellitus**
- **Alcohol**
- **B12 deficiency**
- Chronic kidney disease
- Cancers (lymphoma, multiple myeloma) & paraneoplastic syndromes
- Charcot Marie Tooth Disease (hereditary sensory motor neuropathy)
- **Drugs (Mnemonic: NO IMPACTS):** Nitrofurantoin; Oncovir (Vincristine) & other chemotherapy agents; Isoniazid; Metronidazole; Phenytoin; Amiodarone; Ciprofloxacin & other fluoroquinolones (potentially irreversible); Thalidomide; Statins
- Denervation from accidental injury or surgery
- Endocrine — Hypothyroidism
- Friedrich's ataxia
- Gammopathy of unknown significance (MGUS)
- Heavy Metals (Iron, Lead, Arsenic)
- Inflammation & immune over activity — Connective tissue disorders (RA, SLE, Sjogren's syndrome), Systemic vasculitides (Churg Strauss Syndrome, Wegener's granulomatosis, PAN), Sarcoidosis, Multiple sclerosis.
- Retroviral disease & its treatment (try to avoid using the term HIV).

Motor neuropathy: Guillain-Barre syndrome, Lead toxicity, Porphyria

Sensorimotor: Charcot Marie Tooth Disease (aka Hereditary Sensorimotor Neuropathy).

Mononeuritis multiplex:
Infections: Leprosy (commonest cause worldwide), Lyme Disease
Metabolic: Diabetes
Inflammation: Connective tissue disorders (RA, Lupus, Sjogren's) & systemic vasculitides; Sarcoidosis.
Cancers: Lymphoma
Infiltrative disorders: Amyloidosis

History & Investigations	Management

- History: family history, alcohol consumption and medications; Autonomic symptoms (erectile dysfunction; gastroparesis; constipation; postural hypotension) may co-exist.
- Fasting blood sugar, B12 levels, ESR, Thyroid function tests, autoantibodies
- Nerve conduction studies (usually reduced in demyelinating pathologies like HSMN Type 1 but relatively preserved in axonal degeneration Type 2 HSMN)
- Nerve biopsy
	- MDT approach including PT & OT to maintain independence with ADL.
	- Walking aids/orthoses
	- Treat neuropathic pain with tricyclic antidepressants & anticonvulsants (pregabalin, gabapentin).
	- Orthopaedic surgery to correct deformities.
	- Treat underlying cause if possible.
	
	   ➢ DM — Glycaemic control, lifestyle modifications.
	   ➢ B12 deficiency — Replace B12.
	   ➢ Abstain from alcohol
	   ➢ Stop/Avoid relevant drugs
	   ➢ Hereditary causes — Genetic counselling

4A: Charcot Marie Tooth Disease

Genetics: Autosomal Dominant. PMP 22 gene on Chromosome 17.

Examination: *Examiners might cover lower limbs and ask you to do an upper limb examination. Good exposure is vital. Use the 2W2P method.*

- General examination: Walking aids, Ankle support, Orthoses, Scars.
- Gait: High Stepping; Bilateral Foot drop.
- Upper limbs: Claw hands (hyperextension deformities at MCP and flexion deformities at PIP & DIP joints); Postural Tremor; Distal wasting including small muscles of hand (dorsal guttering); Absent reflexes; Palpable ulnar nerve; 'Gloves' distribution symmetrical sensory loss.
- Lower limbs: Hammer toes, Bilateral Pes cavus & foot drop, Scars from previous corrective surgery *(look closely for scars over neck of fibula as patients with common peroneal nerve injury can have foot drop as well but this is unlikely to be bilateral)*, distal wasting (inverted Champagne bottles), absent ankle jerks, symmetrical distal sensorimotor neuropathy in a 'stocking' distribution, palpable lateral popliteal nerve.
- Offer to do ophthalmoscopy (? Optic atrophy; retinitis pigmentosa).

Pes cavus in PACES: This is an important sign. Think about the following conditions the moment you pick it up. **New onset pes cavus warrants investigation for cord tumours. ALWAYS EXAMINE THE SPINE.**

Bilateral	Unilateral
<ul><li>Charcot Marie Tooth Disease</li><li>Friedrich's Ataxia</li><li>Muscular dystrophies</li><li>Hereditary spastic paraparesis</li><li>Syringomyelia</li></ul>	<ul><li>Poliomyelitis</li><li>Spinal cord tumours & trauma</li></ul>

4B: Common Peroneal Nerve Palsy

Clinical Examination

- General examination: Walking aids, Ankle support, Orthoses, Scars.
- Gait: High Stepping; Unilateral foot drop.
- Lower limbs: Orthopaedic surgery scars (over neck of fibula/ previous knee surgery); Unable to dorsiflex or evert ankle; Unable to dorsiflex big toe; ANKLE INVERSION PRESERVED (if lost think about L5 Radiculopathy); Preserved ankle jerk (RULES OUT MOTOR NEUROPATHIES); Sensory loss over dorsum of foot sparing 5th toe.

Discussion: Aetiology, Differentiation from L5 radiculopathy, Management

Cause:

- Trauma (# fibula, after knee surgery)
- External compression,
- Part of Mononeuritis multiplex.

Why is this not an L5 Radiculopathy? ANKLE INVERSION IS PRESERVED. In L5 radiculopathy, hip abduction and ankle inversion are lost and loss of sensation extends further proximally up the lateral side of the leg. SLR test is positive.

Investigations: Clinical diagnosis. However, neurophysiology and EMG are useful. MRI lumbar spine can help exclude an L5 lesion if in doubt.

Management: Supportive. As above + treatment of cause.

Case 5: Myasthenia Gravis

Clinical Examination: You might be asked to examine cranial nerves (complex ophthalmoplegia), limbs (proximal myopathy) or to examine patient neurologically. The key is in picking up the **ptosis** and generalised lethargy on inspection. With cranial nerves, once the complex ophthalmoplegia is discovered, proceed to demonstrate fatiguability & proximal myopathy. Use the screening techniques in the 2W2P method with the limbs.

Classical Signs	Additional Signs
• General inspection: Bilateral ptosis (*can be unilateral as well*), myasthenic snarl (horizontal smile with bilateral facial weakness). • Screening: Fatiguability (30 to 1), nasal speech. • Cranial nerves: Complex ophthalmoplegia, diplopia • Don't forget to offer to do ophthalmoscopy. • Limbs: Proximal myopathy (upper limbs > lower limbs).	• Thymectomy scar. • Evidence of other autoimmune disease: • Diabetes — finger-prick marks, insulin injection site lipodystrophy, insulin pens/pumps. • RA — symmetrical deforming polyarthropathy involving small hand joints. • Hyper/hypothyroidism (St 2 & 5) • Lupus — rashes, arthropathy. • Immunosuppressive therapy.

Sample Presentation: On neurological examination of this young woman, I note the presence of a myasthenic snarl and bilateral ptosis worsened by activity and sustained vertical up gaze & improved by rest. Fatiguability was demonstrated by worsening clarity of speech and increasing nasal intonation with prolonged vocalisation. The patient's jaw & neck dropped with prolonged vocalisation. Examination of the cranial nerves reveals bilateral complex ophthalmoplegia, diplopia and bilateral facial muscle weakness. Examination of upper limbs revealed proximal myopathy with fatiguability. Sensation & reflexes were preserved. There were no obvious signs of other autoimmune disease. To complete my examination, I would like to perform ophthalmoscopy & a formal assessment of hearing to rule out mitochondrial myopathies. A full history is needed to proceed including drug history (to rule out drug induced myasthenic syndrome) and past medical history of pulmonary neoplasms *(avoid using the term cancer in front of the patient)*.

Common Discussion topics: Pathophysiology, Lambert Eaton Myasthenic syndrome, Investigations, Management.

Investigations	Management
• Anti nAChR (90 % cases) • Anti-MuSK • EMG (decremented response to stimuli) • Tensilon test — Improved symptoms with edrophonium; false positives include MND, GBS, Lambert Eaton myasthenic syndrome; risk of cardiac complications • MRI/CT Mediastinum to rule out thymoma • Additional tests to screen for other autoimmune disease (TFT, BM, Autoimmune screen)	• DON'T FORGET GENERAL MEASURES (MDT Approach, Education) • Symptomatic management with anticholinesterase inhibitor (Pyridostigmine). • Immunomodulatory therapy – Rapid — IVIG, Plasmapheresis Long term — Steroids & steroid sparing agents. • Surgery — Thymectomy. • Myasthenic crises should be managed in HDU/ITU with close monitoring of respiratory function.

Pathophysiology: Autoimmune disorder characterised by antibodies against post synaptic membrane nicotinic acetylcholine receptors (nAchR) at neuromuscular junctions with impaired signal transmission secondary to accelerated complement mediated destruction & functional blockage of AChR. Associated with thymomas (10 %) & other autoimmune disorders including thyroid disease (10 %).

Epidemiology: Prevalence of 20/100,000 (male: female = 1:2). Female predominance when presenting in the $2^{nd}/3^{rd}$ decade of life; male predominance in 6th–8th decades (often misdiagnosed).

Presentation: Ocular complaints in first year, Myasthenic crisis in 20 % cases of generalised myasthenia.

Differential diagnoses: Lambert Eaton Myasthenic syndrome presents with similar symptoms and is associated with small cell Ca lung in 60 % cases. It is characterised by antibodies against pre-synaptic voltage gated Ca channels. It can be differentiated from myasthenia by **improvement of symptoms following exercise with incremental response** to repetitive single nerve stimulation. Proximal myopathy is worse in **lower limbs** & ocular symptoms are rare. Treatment involves supportive treatment, Amifampridine (contraindicated in LQTS, Epilepsy, Asthma) and treating the Ca lung.

Drugs that exacerbate myasthenia:

- Antibiotics (Macrolides, Quinolones, Aminoglycosides, Tetracyclines)
- Antidysrhythmic (CCB, Beta blockers, Lignocaine, Procainamide)
- Antipsychotics (Phenothiazine's, Atypical antipsychotics)
- Antiepileptic (Phenytoin)
- Mood stabilisers (Lithium)
- Steroids can paradoxically worsen myasthenia for up to 10/7 in 15 % cases with subsequent improvement.

Bilateral complex ophthalmoplegia:

- Grave's ophthalmopathy
- Myasthenia gravis
- Miller Fisher syndrome (Ataxia, Areflexia, Ophthalmoplegia; variant of GBS)
- Kearns-Sayre syndrome, a mitochondrial myopathy which is a severe variant of Chronic progressive external ophthalmoplegia (CPEO); assoc. with ptosis, ophthalmoplegia, pigmentary retinopathy, deafness, DM, AV conduction defects, cerebellar ataxia).

Case 6: Absent Ankle Jerk With Extensor Plantars

This finding implies a combination of upper and lower motor neuron lesions and differential diagnoses include:

- Motor Neuron Disease/Amyotrophic lateral sclerosis
- Friedrich's Ataxia
- Subacute combined degeneration of the cord
- Cauda Equina & Conus medullaris syndromes
- Demyelination/Multiple Sclerosis
- Taboparesis/Neurosyphilis
- Pellagra
- Other causes of peripheral neuropathy (especially diabetes) in combination with cord pathology can make diagnosis challenging and must always be ruled out.

In this section we shall focus on MND, Friedrich's ataxia and Subacute Combined Degeneration of the cord, which are commonly evaluated in the examination.

6A — Motor Neuron Disease

Clinical Examination		Investigations
\multicolumn{2}{c}{Inspection}	NO SPECIFIC DIAGNOSTIC TESTS.
\multicolumn{2}{l}{Walking aids; Ankle support/orthoses for foot drop; Wasting, fasciculation. **NO SCARS ON THE SPINE** (*diagnosis is questionable if present*), Drooling.}	**EMG** — fasciculation. **NERVE CONDUCTION STUDY** — axonal degeneration. **NEUROIMAGING** (MRI) to rule out main differential diagnoses:
\multicolumn{2}{c}{Cranial Nerves}	• Cervical myelopathy
Bulbar palsy	Pseudobulbar palsy	• Cord compression
Donald Duck Speech Nasal speech; difficulty with consonants. Atrophic tongue; Fasciculation Normal jaw jerk	**'Hot potato speech'** Stiff spastic tongue. Brisk jaw jerk. UMN signs elsewhere.	• Syringomyelia
		Management
		• MDT approach & Symptomatic treatment:
\multicolumn{2}{c}{*Oculomotor Muscles Preserved. No Sensory Loss.*}	✓ Dysphagia — Dietician, PEG. ✓ Dysarthria — SLT.
\multicolumn{2}{c}{Upper & Lower Limbs}	✓ Pain — Analgesia, Pain team input, Palliative care.
\multicolumn{2}{l}{Mixed UMN + LMN signs in a variable pattern. Classically, UMN signs in LL, and LMN signs in UL.}	✓ Mobility issues — PT, OT, Orthoses/Walking aids. ✓ Secretions — Anticholinergic drugs, Hyoscine patches.
	UMN	LMN	
Tone	Spastic	Flaccid	✓ Spasticity — Baclofen
Power	Reduced	Reduced	✓ Respiratory failure — NIV
Reflexes	Brisk Hoffman's sign — UL Extensor plantars — LL	Absent	• Early specialist input incl. palliative care. • Patient education. • Respect patient's autonomy & wishes. • Riluzole (Glutamate antagonist) 3-month increase in survival. • Edravone (free radical scavenger for ALS < 2 years or advanced disease; FVC ≥ 80 %).
Sensation	PRESERVED		
Coordination	PRESERVED		

NB. With unilateral cranial nerve lesions in bulbar palsy, the uvula deviates to the side away from lesion and tongue is pulled towards the side of lesion.

Common Discussion Topics: Differentials, Investigations, Management.

During your examination, examine the part of the nervous system you were asked to examine first, e.g. cranial nerves. After completing this, once you have demonstrated relevant signs, proceed to examine the parts of the neurological examination not done, e.g. upper/lower limbs. If you run out of time, mention what you would look for in those examinations in your presentation.

Sample Presentations: Start with, "On neurological examination of this patient, I note the presence of walking aids on the bedside. There are **NO VISIBLE SCARS ON THE SPINE.**

A) The patient had dysarthria & dysphonia with a nasal speech lacking in modulation. The extraocular muscles were preserved. There is a lower motor neuron type of facial weakness with loss of forehead creasing. There was palatal paralysis with a wasted tongue and prominent fasciculations. The jaw jerk was absent. These features are consistent with a bulbar palsy. Further neurological examination of the upper & lower limbs revealed....

B) Examination of the upper limbs reveals there was generalised wasting including of small muscles of the hands with claw hand deformities, prominent fasciculations, hypertonia and hyperreflexia with preserved sensation & coordination. Further neurological examination of the cranial nerves & lower limbs revealed....

C) Examination of the lower limbs reveals wasting, prominent fasciculations, brisk knee jerk with absent ankle jerk & extensor plantars with ankle clonus. Sensation & coordination are preserved. Further neurological examination of the upper limbs & cranial nerves revealed....

Then say... "With preserved coordination & sensation, these features are consistent with MND. I would proceed to take a full history including onset, duration & progression of symptoms, past medical history of spinal cord injury and proceed with neuroimaging to rule out my differential diagnoses of cord compression, cervical myelopathy & syringomyelia.

Different forms of MND:

- ✓ Amyotrophic lateral sclerosis: UMN + LMN signs. Spastic paraparesis.
- ✓ Progressive muscular atrophy: LMN signs. Anterior horn cells affected.
- ✓ Primary lateral sclerosis: UMN signs.
- ✓ Progressive bulbar palsy: Worst prognosis. Lower cranial nerves & suprabulbar nuclei of IX, X, XII'th cranial nerves.

Causes of bulbar & pseudobulbar palsy:

Bulbar Palsy	Pseudobulbar Palsy
Degenerative: • Amyotrophic lateral sclerosis • Syringobulbia Autoimmune: • Myasthenia gravis Inflammation/Infections: • GBS • Polio • Lyme disease • Neurosarcoidosis Tumours: Lower Brainstem Metabolic: Central pontine myelinosis Vascular: Medullary infarction Congenital/Rare causes: • Kennedy's disease (spinal & bulbar muscular atrophy) • Acute intermittent porphyria	Trauma: Head injury Metabolic: Wilson's disease; Osmotic demyelination syndrome Toxins: Nitrous oxide use Tumours: High brainstem Infarction: Bilateral cortical strokes, CADASIL syndrome. Degenerative: • MND • Parkinson's disease • Multisystem atrophy • Progressive supranuclear palsy Demyelination

6B — Friedrich's Ataxia

Definition & pathophysiology: Autosomal recessive trinucleotide repeat disorder (GAA) on chromosome 9q13 (FRATAXIN gene). Neurodegenerative condition affecting Posterior Columns, Corticospinal tracts & Cerebellum.

Clinical examination: Work your way down; bilateral symmetrical signs.

- General examination: Young patient, Wheelchair, Walking aids, Orthoses.
- Speech: Dysarthria (West Register Street)
- Eyes: Nystagmus, Saccades
- Mouth: High arched palate
- Spine: Kyphoscoliosis
- Upper limbs: Bilateral dysdiadochokinesia, intention tremor, ataxic handshake, past pointing, hyporeflexia.
- Lower limbs: **Pes cavus, Hammer toes**, Scars from corrective foot surgery, Distal wasting, Dorsal column signs (Proprioception & vibration lost; Romberg's +ve), Ataxic gait, Absent ankle jerk, Extensor Plantars.
- Check for complications: Heart sounds & murmurs (HOCM; 50 %); Pulse & ECG (AV conduction defect); Urine dips & BM (10 % have diabetes); Ophthalmoscopy — Optic atrophy (30%); Sensorineural hearing loss (10 %); History of bladder dysfunction.

Discussion: Pathophysiology, Genetics, Investigations, Management.

Presentation: Follow Case 3. Present obvious deformities first.

Investigations: Family history, Nerve conduction studies & biopsy, Rule out MS (MRI, CSF oligoclonal bands), Genetic studies.

Management: MDT approach to maintain independence with ADLs; PT; OT; Ankle foot orthoses; Orthopaedic foot surgery; Treatment of complications (visual aids/hearing aids/treat diabetes & cardiac complications); Genetic counselling (Siblings of affected individual have a 25% chance of being affected, 50% chance of being an asymptomatic carrier, and 25% chance of having no pathogenic variant. Warn about anticipation).

6C — Subacute Combined Degeneration of the Cord

Clinical Examination

Classical Signs	Additional Signs
• Dorsal column signs: Loss of vibration & proprioception. Sensory ataxia (Romberg's sign is positive) • Light touch is lost but pain and temperature (spinothalamic tract) are usually preserved. • Pyramidal tract signs: Brisk knee jerk but absent ankle jerk (lost due to peripheral neuropathy) and extensor plantars.	• Inflamed tongue, Anaemia (conjunctival pallor). • Evidence of other autoimmune disease (Thyroid disorders & Diabetes are associated with pernicious anaemia). • Abdomen: Splenomegaly, Previous gastrectomy scars.

Sample Presentation: On examination of the lower limbs, this young patient has a positive Romberg's test, suggestive of sensory ataxia. Tone and power are preserved. The knee jerk is brisk, but the ankle jerk is lost with extensor plantars. There is loss of light touch, vibration and proprioception. Pain & temperature sensations are preserved. In absence of cerebellar symptoms & pes cavus, my differential diagnoses would include demyelination & subacute combined degeneration of the cord. Diabetes in combination with cord pathology can produce similar symptoms and must be ruled out.

Common Discussion topics: Differential diagnoses, Causes of peripheral neuropathy & B12 deficiency, Investigations, Management.

Investigations	Management
• FBC & MCV (macrocytosis), • Reticulocyte count • Haematinics (B12, Folate, Ferritin) • Parietal cell Ab & intrinsic factor • OGD with D2 biopsies • MRI spine • HbA1c/Blood Glucose • CSF oligoclonal bands	• MDT approach. • Patient education. • PT/OT/Orthotics — maintain independence with ADLs. • B12 replacement tends to improve sensory symptoms more than motor symptoms.

Note: Lhermitte's phenomenon is common to both demyelination & subacute combined degeneration of cord.

Differential diagnoses would include

- Demyelination
- Friedrich's ataxia (pes cavus, cerebellar signs)
- Taboparesis and
- Combination of peripheral neuropathy (e.g. diabetes) with cervical myelopathy.

Causes of B12 deficiency (common in the UK; 6 % aged < 60 years and up to 20 % in those over 60 years):

1. Dietary deficiency: Especially vegan diets.
2. Atrophic gastritis: H. pylori, Advancing age, Pernicious anaemia (Autoimmune metaplastic atrophic gastritis)
3. Parasites: Fish tapeworm
4. Drugs: OCP, Ibuprofen, Colchicine, PPI, Cimetidine, Metformin, Antiepileptic medications.
5. Gastric bypass surgery
6. Ileostomy
7. Tropical sprue
8. Nitrous oxide (2nd most common recreational drug in the UK after marijuana in young adults aged 16–years).

Case 7: Syringomyelia

Clinical Examination: Use the 2W2P method.

Classical Signs	Additional Signs
Inspection	Horner's syndrome: Remember *PAMELa*
Charcot joints (especially elbows)	Partial ptosis
Distal wasting & weakness including wasting of small muscles of hands.	Anhidrosis
Fasciculations in upper limbs.	Miosis
Screening	Enophthalmos
Kyphoscoliosis	Loss of ciliary reflex
Midline spinal scar (from previous laminectomies or syrinx decompression).	Bulbar palsy: If lower cranial nerves involved (syringobulbia)
Examination proper	
At the level: Anterior horn cells — LMN signs Dissociated sensory loss (decussating spinothalamic tracts affected, dorsal columns preserved) Below the level: UMN signs below the syrinx (Corticospinal tracts) Usually asymmetrical	

	UL	LL
Tone	Flaccid	Spastic
Power	Distal weakness	Pyramidal
Reflexes	Absent deep tendon reflexes	Brisk tendon reflexes, plantars extensor
Coordination	Preserved	
Sensation	Pain and temperature lost; vibration and position normal	Usually preserved

Understanding syringomyelia: A fluid filled gliosis lined cavity within the spinal cord, usually between C2 and T9. It can expand in diameter and length, ascend to the brainstem (when it is called syringobulbia) and descend further downwards. As it grows, there is progressive, asymmetric neurological decline.

Pathophysiology: CSF blockage, Spinal cord injury, Intramedullary spinal tumours, Idiopathic. Causes include:

- *Congenital malformations*: Arnold Chiari malformation type 1 (commonest; lower part of brain extends into spinal canal); Klippel Feil syndrome (cervical vertebral fusion at birth); tethered cord syndrome.

- *Acquired*: After spinal cord trauma, tumours, infections & inflammation (transverse myelitis, demyelination).

Sample Presentation: On neurological examination of the upper limbs there are Charcot deformities of elbow joints, prominent fasciculations, kyphoscoliosis and a midline surgical spinal scar. I note the presence of painless scars & ulcers over the digits with callosities over the knuckles. There is asymmetrical hypotonia associated with absent deep tendon reflexes and loss of light touch and temperature with preserved sense of position & vibration in the upper limbs. The sensation returns to normal at the level of T10 *(TRY TO FIND THE LOWER LEVEL OF THE SYRINX)*. Examination of lower limbs reveals spastic gait, hypertonia, and brisk tendon reflexes. The combination of LMN signs in UL with UMN signs in LL with diffuse sensory loss and Charcot joints in elbows is in keeping with a diagnosis of syringomyelia. The cervical scar suggests surgical repair of a syrinx. Further history should be guided towards onset, duration & progression of symptoms including neuropathic pain & excessive sweating. Further neuroimaging is needed to rule out spinal pathology.

Common Discussion topics: Differential diagnoses, investigations & management.

Differential Diagnoses

- Brainstem & Cord pathologies (trauma, tumour, infection, infarction, demyelination)
- Guillan Barre Syndrome (usually lower limbs affected first)
- Motor neuron disease (no sensory loss).

Investigations	Management
MRI spine	MDT approach (PT, OT, SW)
Myelography (± HRCT) may be useful if MRI not available	Patient education
	Neuro Rehab
Neurophysiology (low amplitude & delayed responses in myelopathy)	No medical treatment
	Surgical options:
LP to rule out CSF oligoclonal bands & Albumino-cytological dissociation	Cervical decompression
	Dorsolateral myelotomy
	Shunt formation
	• Syringoperitoneal shunt
	• Syringosubarachnoid shunt
	• Ventriculoperitoneal shunt

Case 8: Spastic Paraparesis

Clinical Examination

Classical Signs	Additional Signs
Inspection: • Walking aids • Spinal scars • Pes cavus (if present think about congenital causes; new onset: think cord tumours) • Evidence of self-catheterisation (sphincter disturbance) Screening: Spastic diplegic gait. Examination proper: • Tone: Increased • Power: Reduced • Reflexes: Brisk, upgoing planters • Coordination: If affected think about Friedrich's ataxia, MS • Sensation: Is there a sensory level? Find it. If sensation normal, think about MND.	• Cord trauma/tumour/infection (especially tuberculosis): spinal surgery scars • Demyelination: INO, Optic atrophy, cerebellar signs, diffuse sensory loss with mixed UMN+LMN signs • Friedrich's ataxia: Bilateral Pes Cavus; absent ankle jerk, extensor plantars; ataxic gait; cerebellar signs • Hereditary spastic paraplegia: Bilateral pes cavus, spastic diplegic gait. Spasticity>weakness. • Other signs may/may not be present and includes impaired vision due to cataracts and problems with the optic nerve and retina of the eye, ataxia (lack of muscle coordination; making it clinically difficult to differentiate from Friedrich's), epilepsy, cognitive impairment, peripheral neuropathy, and deafness

Sample Presentation: On neurological examination of the lower limbs, I note walking aids on the bedside. There is bilateral pes cavus with no spinal scars. There is very little muscle wasting. The patient walks with a spastic diplegic gait. There are no spinal scars and Romberg's test is positive suggestive of sensory ataxia. There is hypertonia with pathologically brisk reflexes in the lower extremities associated with ankle clonus and upgoing planters. There is weakness with ankle dorsiflexion and mild weakness with hip flexion, but individual movements were difficult to examine because of profound spasticity. The reflexes are pathologically brisk with upgoing planters. Heel shin test is negative. There is decreased perception of sharp touch below the knees with some loss of vibration, but light touch & temperature are preserved. In absence of any evidence of neurosurgery and cerebellar signs, the features are consistent with a hereditary spastic paraplegia, but I would like to rule out cord compression, cervical myelopathy and demyelination.

Common Discussion topics: Differential diagnosis, Investigations, Management.

Differential Diagnoses

Congenital	Acquired
• Hereditary spastic paraplegia (Spasticity >>> Weakness in LL) • Friedrich's ataxia	• Cord compression or cervical myelopathy due to spondylosis and **Trauma** (neurosurgery, accidents), **Tumours** (clear sensory level) • **Infection/Inflammation**: Pott's disease (Spinal TB), Transverse myelitis (clear sensory level) • **Infarction**: Anterior spinal artery infarcts • **Demyelination**

Investigations	Management
Tests to rule out structural disease & demyelination: • MRI brain & spinal cord • CSF — oligoclonal bands (MS) • Visual evoked potentials • Genetic testing for congenital conditions.	*"... multidisciplinary approach with early involvement of specialist physicians, physiotherapy, occupational therapy and neurological rehabilitation services with focus on patient & family education. Specific management will depend on the cause."*

Cord compression is a medical emergency and may need urgent neurosurgical intervention to decompress the cord with/without steroids and radiotherapy.

Case 9: Internuclear Ophthalmoplegia

Clinical Examination

Classical Signs	Additional Signs
On lateral gaze: • The abducting eye demonstrates coarse, jerky nystagmus • The adducting eye is slow to or is unable to adduct	Other features of demyelination: • Cerebellar Syndrome • Marcus Gunn Pupil • Spastic Paraparesis • Walking Aids, etc

Sample Presentation: The patient is a young Caucasian female in a wheelchair. Her speech has a slurred, staccato character. Examination of the cranial nerves revealed a jerky nystagmus on the right side on abduction. However, the opposite eye is unable to adduct and the patient reports diplopia. Convergence is preserved. There were no other neurological deficits on examination of the cranial nerves.

I noted an ataxic handshake and further examination of upper limbs reveals a positive rebound phenomenon, intention tremor, past pointing, hypotonia & hyporeflexia worse on the right. I would like to complete my examination by performing a full neurological examination of both upper and lower limbs including gait to look for evidence of ataxia and fundoscopy to check for optic atrophy.

These features are consistent with internuclear ophthalmoplegia suggestive of a medial longitudinal fasciculus lesion as well as a right sided cerebellar lesion. I would like to suggest demyelination as the possible aetiology in view of a combination of INO with cerebellar signs as well as patient's age, sex & ethnicity.

Other differentials include cerebellar trauma, intracranial space occupying lesions (ICSOL) including tumours & abscesses, cerebrovascular events, paraneoplastic syndromes & drugs/toxins including phenytoin and alcohol. A full history of onset, duration, progression and aggravating & relieving factors is needed along with past medical history, drug history, personal history including history of alcohol abuse and a full family history. Further investigations should include neuroimaging to rule out structural brain & cord lesions and to visualise CNS plaques, CSF for oligoclonal bands and EEG for visual evoked potentials.

Demyelination can be evaluated in the examination in several ways. It can be part of a cranial nerve examination where one is expected to pick up one of the following findings and proceed accordingly:

- Optic nerve: Optic atrophy, Marcus Gunn Pupil (RAPD) (Case 10A)
- Internuclear ophthalmoplegia & Diplopia
- Facial nerve weakness (usu. UMN) (Case 10C)
- Cerebellar signs — nystagmus, scanning dysarthria (Case 3)

As part of a neurological examination of limbs where it may present as:

- Cerebellar syndrome (DANISH) (Case 3)
- Mixed lower motor and upper motor signs with non-specific sensory loss (e.g. spastic paraparesis with dorsal column signs ± variable loss of light touch/pin prick) (Case 8).

Presentations: In addition to above features, patients might develop mood disorders and autonomic dysfunction as well. Two classic features include:

- **Uhthoff's phenomenon:** worsening symptoms after hot bath/exercise
- **Lhermitte's sign:** lightening pains in spine on neck flexion

Diagnosis: McDonald's criteria — CNS plaques disseminated in time & space.

Investigations

- MRI Brain & spine to rule out structural brain & cord lesions and to visualise CNS plaques,
- CSF for oligoclonal bands
- EEG for visual evoked potentials.

4 forms of disease:

- Clinically isolated syndrome (CIS)
- Relapsing-remitting MS (RRMS)
- Primary progressive MS (PPMS)
- Secondary progressive MS (SPMS)

Management

Do not forget **general measures** ("... **multidisciplinary approach** with early involvement of **specialist physicians, physiotherapy, occupational therapy, social workers** and **neurological rehabilitation** services with focus on **patient & family education**").

Symptomatic/Supportive management

- **Baclofen** for spasticity
- **Carbamazepine** for neuropathic pain
- Autonomic symptoms/sphincter disturbance — **self catheterisation**

Disease Modifying Treatments

Primary Progressive MS — Monoclonal antibody **Ocrelizumab** (ORTARIO TRIAL; FDA approved in March'17) is the drug of choice. Other medications (**Methylprednisolone, Methotrexate, Cladribine, IVIG** and **Mitoxantrone**) lack in trial evidence in primary progressive disease but can be used in patients intolerant of Ocrelizumab empirically.

Relapsing remitting disease — Pulsed **IV methyl prednisolone** 3/7 shorten duration of acute relapses.

Interferon Beta, Natalizumab & **Glatiramer acetate, Teriflunomide** and **Fingolimod** reduce relapses. **Dimethyl fumarate** can be used orally.

Secondary progressive disease — In these patients, continue DMT from relapsing remitting phase or switch to alternate DMT. Options include:

- **Interferon Beta**
- **IV glucocorticoid pulses** with or without **IV cyclophosphamide** boost
- **Methotrexate**
- **Siponimod** (sphingosine 1-phosphate receptor modulator) reduced the risk of confirmed disability progression at 3 & 6 months as well as reduced 12- and 24-month annualised relapse rates & volume of brain lesions in the EXPAND trial.

Case 10: Cranial Nerve Syndromes

10A — Optic Atrophy & Marcus Gunn Pupil

Clinical Examination

Classical Signs	Additional Signs
• The affected eye dilates instead of contracting when light is shone into it. • Consensual reflex is preserved • Fundoscopy: Pale discs	• Features of demyelination: Cerebellar Syndrome Internuclear ophthalmoplegia Spastic Paraparesis Walking Aids, etc. • Features of Grave's disease & Grave's ophthalmopathy. • Diabetes: Insulin pumps & pens; finger prick BM checking marks; injection sites.

Discussion: Cause, Investigations, Management.

Aetiology:

Retina:

- Central retinal arterial or venous occlusion
- Retinitis pigmentosa
- Tobacco Amblyopia

Optic nerve:

- Glaucoma
- Ischaemic optic atrophy
- Papilloedema
- Optic neuritis (demyelination, infections, connective tissue disease & vasculitis)
- Trauma
- Inherited causes (Friedrich's ataxia, Leber's hereditary OA, Autosomal dominant optic atrophy)
- Compressive features are related to tumours, thyroid eye disease, optic nerve sheath meningioma.

Optic chiasma: Compression from tumours.
Optic tract: Pituitary adenoma.

Others:

- Metabolic causes including Diabetes (can be a part of a mitochondrial disease or on its own), B12 deficiency, Grave's ophthalmopathy
- Toxins: Methanol

Investigations	Management
<ul><li>Rule out structural disease & demyelination: MRI, LP, EEG</li><li>Blood glucose/HbA1c</li><li>TFT/USS thyroid</li><li>Vitamin B12</li><li>Autoimmune screen: ANA, ENA, Anti DS DNA, ANCA, ESR</li><li>Genetic testing (congenital causes)</li></ul>	"... multidisciplinary approach with early involvement of specialist physicians, physiotherapy, occupational therapy and neurological rehabilitation services with focus on patient & family education. Specific management will depend on the cause"

10B — Oculomotor and Abducens Nerve Lesions

Clinical Examination: 3rd NERVE PALSY

Classical Signs	Additional Signs
• Eye 'down and out' • Ptosis • Restriction of movement in all directions except abduction • Pupil spared if medical cause of CN III palsy • Pupil dilated if damage to parasympathetic nerve fibres	• Signs relating to aetiology — e.g. diabetic finger prick marks • Features suggestive of underlying vasculitis • Evidence of surgery for intracranial aneurysm repair

Clinical Examination: 6th NERVE PALSY

Classical Signs	Additional Signs
• Eye is deviated medially • Diplopia on abduction — the outer image disappears when the affected eye is covered.	• Clubbed fingernails (TB) • RAPD (demyelination) • Otitis media in ipsilateral ear (Gradenigo's syndrome)

Discussion: Causes, Investigations, Management.

Quick Revision: SO4 LR6 Rest are 3. Cranial nerve IV supplies the Superior Oblique. Cranial nerve VI supplies the Lateral Rectus. Cranial nerve III supplies the remaining oculomotor muscles.

Causes:

- <u>Brainstem</u>: Vascular lesions; Demyelination; Compressive lesions
- <u>Basal area</u>: Tuberculous infection, infiltration with sarcoid/meningitis, posterior communicating artery aneurysm
- <u>Cavernous sinus/orbit</u>: sepsis, tumours, intracavernous carotid artery aneurysms

- As part of Mononeuritis multiplex: Diabetes, Connective tissue disorders (RA, Lupus, Sjogren's) & systemic vasculitides (esp. Temporal arteritis), Sarcoidosis, Amyloidosis, Certain cancers (lymphomas).

Investigations	Management
- Rule out structural disease & demyelination: MRI, LP, EEG. - Blood glucose/HbA1c - TFT/USS thyroid - Vitamin B12. - Autoimmune screen: ANA, ENA, Anti DS DNA, ANCA, ESR. - Arteriography if pupil involved (3rd nerve palsy)	- General supportive measures - MDT approach - Reassurance - Treatment of cause

10C — Facial Palsy

Clinical Examination

Classical Signs	Additional Signs
- Paralysis of one side of the face - Inability to close eye fully - Drooping mouth - Smooth forehead (due to involvement of frontalis muscle) (LMN lesions) - Smooth nasolabial fold - Eyeballs roll upward on attempted eye closure (Bell's phenomenon)	- Sparing of the upper face (UMN lesion) — look for ipsilateral limb weakness - Loss of taste to the anterior 2/3 of tongue - Loss of salivation/lacrimation - Hyperacusis - Vesicles in the external auditory meatus (Ramsey-Hunt syndrome) - Parotid swellings - Loss of the corneal reflex; Sensorineural hearing loss; Cerebellar signs (cerebellopontine angle lesion)

Causes	Investigations
- Bell's palsy: idiopathic; usually after a viral infection - Ramsay-Hunt syndrome: reactivation of Herpes Zoster in the geniculate nucleus - Trauma - Compressive symptoms from Tumours including cerebellopontine angle lesions - Parotid swellings - Demyelination - Cholesteatoma - Part of mononeuritis multiplex - Bilateral facial nerve palsy: Guillain-Barre syndrome, Neurosarcoid - Lyme's disease	- Bell's palsy diagnosed clinically - Rule out common causes of mononeuritis multiplex if relevant features: Blood glucose/HbA1c TFT/USS thyroid Vitamin B12. Autoimmune screen: ANA, ENA, anti DS DNA, ANCA, ESR. - If cerebellar signs present: Rule out demyelination and structural lesions MRI brain CSF oligoclonal bands - Visual evoked potentials

Case 11: Pupillary Abnormalities

Anisocoria (unequal pupils) can be physiological (20 % of the population). Anisocoria which is worse in bright light (i.e. dilated) include Holmes Adie tonic pupil, 3rd nerve palsy (Case 10B) and pharmacological dilatation (the large pupil is the abnormal pupil). Horner's syndrome and mechanical anisocoria are worse in the dark (the small pupil is the abnormal pupil). A Marcus Gunn pupil (Case 10A) from relative afferent pupillary defect does not cause anisocoria.

11A — Horner's Syndrome

Clinical Examination

Classical Signs (PAMELa)	Additional Signs
• Partial ptosis (Superior tarsal) • Anhidrosis • Miosis (Dilator pupillae) • Enophthalmos (Orbitalis) • Loss of ciliary reflex • Normal extraocular muscles • Normal reaction to light and accommodation	• Cachectic patient • Wasting of the small muscles of the hand • Consolidation (supraclavicular) suggestive of a lung mass • Cervical lymphadenopathy • Thyroid masses • Surgical scars in the neck • Harlequin sign (unilateral sweating after exposure to heat)

Common Discussion topics: Course of the sympathetic pathway; Causes of Horner's Syndrome, Investigations

The sympathetic pathway starts with the first neuron in the hypothalamus and travels through the brainstem, terminating at C8-T1 in the spinal cord. The second neuron (preganglionic) starts at C8-T1 and travels to the superior cervical ganglion. The third neurone travels from the superior cervical ganglion, in proximity to the carotid artery, to the pupil and the upper and lower tarsus muscles.

Site of Lesion & Causes		
Central/1st order neuron (anhidrosis of face, arm and trunk; all the **S**s)	Preganglionic/2nd order neurons (anhidrosis of face only; all the **T**s)	Post ganglionic/3rd order neurons (no anhidrosis limited to forehead; all the **C**s)
• Brainstem **S**trokes • **S**yringomyelia • Multiple **S**clerosis • Encephalitis	• Pancoast's **T**umour • **T**raction of cervical rib on stellate ganglion • **T**hyroid mass • **T**rauma including complications of neck surgery • **T**horacic artery aneurysm	• **C**arotid artery aneurysms & dissections • **C**arotid body tumours • **C**avernous sinus thrombosis • **C**luster headache + Horner's syndrome = Horton's headache

Investigations	Management
• CXR — will identify a neoplastic lesion, cervical rib • CT head/chest • Carotid angiography	• General supportive measures • Treatment of cause

11B — Adie's Tonic Pupil

Clinical Examination: A**DI**e's pupil = **DI**lated

Classical Signs	Additional Signs
• Dilated, irregular pupil • Pupil reacts sluggishly to light • Responds well to accommodation.	Holmes-Adie syndrome: • Middle-aged female patient • Areflexia • Autonomic features (hypohidrosis, postural hypotension, diarrhoea)

Note: During accommodation, normally the pupil constricts to increase depth of focus. If a strong light stimulus is used, the pupils contract to a very small size, returning to its former size very slowly when the stimulus is removed (myotonic pupil). This means that in the examination you might not have time to demonstrate accommodation afterwards. **If you see an abnormal pupil in the exam, always check accommodation before shining a light in the eye.**

Definition: Holmes Adie Syndrome is a benign condition due to damage to the parasympathetic fibres in the ciliary ganglion usually after a bacterial/viral infection characterised by myotonic pupil, areflexia and autonomic neuropathy in middle aged females.

Management: Usually no further investigations needed, and patient should be reassured.

11C — Argyll Robertson Pupil

Clinical Examination

Classical Signs	Additional Signs
• Bilateral small irregular pupil • Argyll Robertson Pupil — **ARP** = **A**ccommodation **R**eflex **P**resent and if reversed; **PRA** = **P**upillary **R**eflex **A**bsent	• Clubbed fingernails (Sarcoid) • Cerebellar syndrome/spastic paraparesis (MS) • Early diastolic murmur (tertiary syphilis) • Fingertip — skinprick marks (Diabetes)

Common Discussion topics: Differential diagnoses: Other causes of light near dissociation (i.e. pupils that accommodate but do not react).

- Perinaud's syndrome aka Dorsal midbrain syndrome is characterised by light near dissociation and VERTICAL GAZE PALSY. The causes include cerebral tumours, strokes and demyelination.
- Adie's syndrome (see previous case) involves DILATED pupils that react sluggishly to light but accommodate well.

With the advent of antibiotics, Argyll Robertson Pupil associated with neurosyphilis is rare in the developed world. Other causes include Diabetes, Demyelination, Neurosarcoidosis and Lyme disease. Although the pathophysiology is not clear it is postulated that bilateral damage to the pretectal nuclei might be responsible.

Case 12: Hemiplegia

Clinical Examination

Classical Signs	Additional Signs
Inspection: • Walking aids, NG tube, PEG • Arm flexed at elbow, pronated • Leg extended at hip and knee • Scars from neurosurgery • Wasting on affected side Screening: • Circumduction gait. • Pronator drift. Examination proper: • Tone: Spastic • Power: Reduced • Brisk reflexes; upgoing plantars • Coordination: If affected think about MS, posterior circulation strokes; Can be affected by weakness. • Sensation lost on the same side in any of the four modalities.	• May have ipsilateral UMN seventh nerve palsy • Speech defects • Homonymous hemianopia/sensory inattention • Look for AF/carotid bruits

Discussion: What territory is affected? Causes of hemiplegia? Investigations. Management.

Aetiology of hemiplegia: Can use the modified surgical sieve if you are stuck (*TrAuMA, Tumour, Infection, Infarction, Demyelination*). Infarction/Haemorrhage are the commonest cause. ICSOL (Intracranial space occupying lesion — tumour/infection e.g. brain abscess), trauma and demyelination can also cause hemiplegic symptoms.

History & Investigations	Management

• PMH of cardiovascular risk factors, previous vascular events, arrhythmias and family history
• Blood pressure
• Blood glucose/HbA1c
• FBC, Coagulation, Lipid profile
• 12 lead ECG (rule out arrhythmias incl. AF)
• Lipid profile
• CXR: cardiomegaly, aspiration
• Echocardiogram (rule out structural heart disease)
• Holter monitoring if arrhythmias suspected
• Carotid Dopplers
• Rule out ICSOL & demyelination if vascular event ruled out: MRI, LP, EEG.
• Vasculitis screen in young patients.
	• MDT approach
	• Specialist physician input
	• Admission to stroke unit
	• PT, OT, Neuro Rehab
	• Patient & family education
	• Treatment of cause
	• Specific treatment of CVAs:
	
	✓ Address cardiovascular risk factors for secondary prevention of strokes:
	    Statins for hypercholesterolaemia
	    Antihypertensives
	    Treat diabetes
	
	✓ Endovascular thrombectomy where available within 8 hours
	✓ Thrombolysis if appropriate within 3 hours (4.5 hours for posterior circulation strokes).
	✓ Aspirin 300 mg 2/52 then Clopidogrel 75 mg OD for 1 year for ischaemic stroke
	✓ Anticoagulation for AF
	✓ Carotid endarterectomy if ≥ 70 % stenosis in ipsilateral internal carotid artery

Using NOACs for AF after stroke: The optimal time at which to start anticoagulation after cerebrovascular events secondary to atrial fibrillation depends on individual risk factors for haemorrhagic transformation of the acute infarct, such as infarct size. The 1 — 3 — 6 — 12 day rule (also known as Diener's rule) has been advocated by some.

- TIAs after day 1.
- Small, nondisabling infarct after 3/7.
- Moderate stroke after 6/7.
- Large infarcts, especially those involving the anterior circulation should not be treated before 12/7, i.e. approximately 2 weeks have elapsed, although most physicians will wait longer before starting anticoagulation.

STATION 4B: ABDOMEN

Introduction

This is probably the easiest of the stations you're going to be examined on. Unless you are terribly unlucky and get a case of a normal abdomen/no clear peripheral signs of disease, the three cases that are most likely to come up are Chronic Liver Disease, a Renal Abdomen and Splenomegaly. The diagnosis will usually be quite evident from peripheral stigmata of hepatic or renal disease. Occasionally there might be vague or unclear clinical signs. Therefore, as in every other station, it is important to be honest about your clinical findings and not make up signs as that is the easiest way to fail this station. In fact, as far as PACES is concerned, **if you are unsure about a sign, we would recommend you do not comment on it, as you might get a 'Borderline' pass and still salvage a point from the examiners if you miss something but if you invent a sign, you will be failed.**

A simple tool to use during the abdominal examination is provided.

- A — Asterixis
- B — Bruising
- C — Clubbing
- D — Dupuytren's contracture
- E — Erythema (palmar)
- F — Fistulae and Finger prick marks for DM, Fetor hepaticus
- G — Gum hypertrophy (Ciclosporin), Gynaecomastia & GCS (impaired in hepatic/metabolic encephalopathy)
- H — Hyperpigmentation (for haemochromatosis) & Hair distribution
- I — 'Eye' — AJAX — see below
- J — Jaundice
- K — Koilonychia
- L — Lymph nodes (*sit the patient up to feel cervical nodes and use this opportunity to inspect the back*).

When examining the eyes, look for AJAX

- A — anaemia
- J — jaundice
- A — arcus senilis
- X — xanthelasma

Then look for spider angiomas (face, upper chest and back are common sites) and move to the abdomen examination proper (inspection, palpation, percussion, auscultation). Common mistakes that people make during the abdominal exam include not sitting down when feeling the abdomen and forgetting to roll the patient to the right when you don't feel a spleen.

Finish off by mentioning examination of external genitalia, hernial orifices, digital rectal examination and urine dipstick.

Case 1: Patient on Renal Replacement Therapy

Clinical Examination

Classical Signs	Additional Signs
• Rutherford Morrison scar in iliac fossa • Fullness underlying scar (**Please be gentle** when feeling transplants. Gentle superficial palpation to feel an unevenness underneath the scar is the best method to feel a transplant. Deep palpation is much less useful. Remember 'Primum non nocere' — First, do no harm). • Bruit • Features of renal replacement therapy — Tenckhoff catheter scars, AV fistulae, Vascath scars.	• An additional upper abdominal scar in a young patient with signs of diabetes might suggest simultaneous Pancreatic and Renal transplantation for diabetic nephropathy. • There might be more than one renal transplantation. Look closely at the scars — Are there multiple scars? The expert surgeon might try to hide a scar within a scar. Is there a scar on each side? • In an Afro-Caribbean patient, think about Lupus and look for the signs.
Signs Suggestive of Aetiology	**Signs of Immunomodulatory Therapy**
• DIABETIC NEPHROPATHY — finger prick marks from blood glucose checks, insulin pens/pumps, cataracts, diabetic dermopathy, necrobiosis lipoidica, lipodystrophy in injection sites, vitiligo (other autoimmune diseases) • HYPERTENSIVE NEPHROPATHY — check BP • ADPKD — ballotable kidneys & nephrectomy scar • VASCULITIDES/ANALGESIC OR DRUG INDUCED NEPHROPATHY — stigmata of connective tissue disease, rashes. • ALPORT'S SYNDROME — hearing aids • TUBEROUS SCLEROSIS — Shagreen patches, Adenoma sebaceum, Subungual fibromas.	• Steroids: Cushingoid facies, back hump, hirsutism, thin bruised skin with purple striae, wasted legs (lemon on matchstick appearance). • Cyclosporin: Gum hypertrophy, Coarse tremor • Tacrolimus: Tremor, Diabetes • Skin cancer removal scars

Six points to mention in the presentation:

- The patient has end stage renal disease on RRT as evidenced by...
- I would like to suggest an aetiology of...
- There is evidence of previous renal replacement therapy as evidenced by...
- The patient is currently receiving renal replacement therapy by...
- They are affiliated with immunomodulatory therapy as evidenced by...
- There is evidence of complications of CKD such as anaemia, hypertension etc.

Sample Presentation

This patient has end stage renal disease as evidenced by the presence of a Rutherford Morrison Scar in the right iliac region with underlying fullness. There is evidence of previous RRT as evidenced by multiple AV fistulae in the antecubital fossae, as well as previous scars of peritoneal dialysis in the abdomen (usually in the iliac region with a small horizontal scar just under the umbilicus) and/or Vascath scars in the upper chest/neck. I would like to suggest an aetiology of ... (*mention differential diagnoses such as DM, HTN, Glomerulonephritides, ADPKD etc*) based on evidence of ... (*e.g. finger pricks for diabetes/bimanually palpable masses or nephrectomy scars for ADPKD*). The patient is receiving RRT by a functional transplant as the fistulae have not been needled recently*. There is evidence of immunomodulatory therapy as evidenced by gum hypertrophy (Ciclosporin)/Cushingoid appearance (Steroids)/Tremor (Tacrolimus)/Scars of skin cancer removal (Tacrolimus/Azathioprine).

*NO BUTTON HOLES — Please make sure you see this during your preparation; the transplant is unlikely to be functional if there is evidence of recent button holes or a Vascath/Tenckhoff catheter.

Discussion: Differential diagnoses, Investigations, Management, Complications.

Most likely causes:

- Diabetic nephropathy
- Glomerulonephritides
- Hypertensive nephropathy
- Autosomal Dominant Polycystic Kidney Disease
- Other causes including obstructive uropathy, amyloidosis, paraproteinaemia, reflux nephropathy and drugs including NSAIDs.

Relevant Investigations	Management
• Urine: Glucose, 24-hour protein, Protein: Creatinine Ratio, Haematuria, Microscopy for casts • Bloods for FBC, Ca, PTH, Serum electrophoresis, Autoimmune screen, Complement, Cryoglobulins, Viral markers (CMV, Hep C) • Imaging: USS KUB • Renal biopsy	• General principles: MDT approach, Early specialist intervention, Patient Education, Dietician and Specialist nurse input, Control hypertension, treat anaemia, PO_4 binders, Renal Diet, Vitamin D supplementation • RRT (Haemodialysis, Peritoneal dialysis, Transplantation). • Management of complications including secondary and tertiary hyperparathyroidism

Indications for acute haemodialysis: The Vowels.

- A — Acidosis
- E — Electrolyte disorders
- I — Intoxicants
- O — Fluid Overload
- U — Uraemic symptoms

Problems following transplantation: Remember the mnemonic **GARLIC**

- **G**raft dysfunction
- **A**cute or chronic rejection
- **R**ecurrence of original disease
- **L**ymphoproliferative disease
- **I**nfections (CMV, PCP) and **I**mmunosuppressant drug toxicity
- **C**ancers (skin, haematological) and **C**ardiovascular disease (hypertension, hyperlipidaemia).

Supplementary Case: Autosomal Dominant Polycystic Kidney Disease

Presentation

- Recurrent urinary tract infections, haematuria, abdominal pain and mass, hypertension.
- Family history of ESRD/ADPKD, strokes (associated with Berry aneurysms), mitral valve prolapse.

Clinical signs: Beware the young patient with the apparently normal abdomen. Are the kidneys palpable?

- Ballotable/palpable kidneys — might feel uneven or cystic, move downwards with respiration; resonant percussion notes (You may be asked how to differentiate from the spleen).
- Polycythaemia (secondary to increased erythropoiesis); Hepatomegaly.
- Signs of renal replacement therapy (AV fistulae/Tunnelled lines/Transplant)
- Signs of CKD — Pallor (anaemia), Pigmentation, Hypertension
- Dipstick the urine for protein and blood.

Genetics

- ADPKD 1 — Chromosome **16** (associated with tuberous sclerosis) (REMEMBER THERE'S A **1** IN **16**)
- ADPKD 2 — Chromosome 4.

Diagnostic Criteria

- At least 2 cysts in 1 kidney or 1 cyst in each kidney in an at-risk patient ≤30-years
- At least 2 cysts in each kidney in an at-risk patient aged 30–59 years
- At least 4 cysts in each kidney for an at-risk patient aged 60 years or older

Treatment

- Monitor renal function and blood pressure.
- Treatment of UTIs and cyst infections usually with gyrase inhibitors (ciprofloxacin, chloramphenicol, clindamycin). The use of Co-Trimoxazole in patients taking Angiotensin Converting Enzyme Inhibitors (ACEI) is not recommended due to risk of hyperkalaemia. Check local protocols.
- Genetic counselling & family screening.
- ACEI: The HALT PKD trial showed a modest but significant reduction in annual increase in renal volume in patients aged 15–49 years with early polycystic kidney disease (EGFR >90) with intensive control of blood pressure. However, combining A2RB with ACEIs did not show an advantage over ACEI alone.
- Tolvaptan (V2 receptor antagonist) slows progression of cyst development & renal insufficiency in adults with CKD stage 1–3 with rapidly progressing disease.

Unilateral Palpable Kidney	Bilateral Palpable Kidney
- ADPKD - Obstructive uropathy/Hydronephrosis (obstruction located proximal to the bladder) - RCC (renal cell cancer)	- ADPKD - Hydronephrosis (bilateral) (obstruction typically located at level of bladder and distal) - RCC (rare; 5 %) - Tuberous sclerosis - Amyloidosis

Case 2: Patient With Chronic Liver Disease

Clinical Examination

Classical Signs

General examination:
- Age, sex, ethnicity
- Body build
- Fetor hepaticus
- Colour of skin (yellow/slate grey)

Hands:
- Asterixis
- Bruising
- Clubbing
- Dupuytren's Contracture
- Erythema (Palmar)
- Leukonychia

Eyes:
- Icterus
- Xanthelasma & arcus senilis (NASH)
- Kayser–Fleischer rings (copper in Descemet's membrane)

Chest/Back/Shoulders:
- Spider naevi
- Gynaecomastia
- Paucity of body hair

Abdomen:
- Ascites (might make other organomegaly difficult to demonstrate)
- Hepatomegaly (smooth/nodular)
- Splenomegaly
- Caput medusa
- Scars (including recent ascitic taps; liver biopsy)
- Testicular atrophy *(you will not be expected to demonstrate this)*.

Lower limbs: Peripheral oedema

Signs Suggestive of Aetiology
• **Alcohol** — unkempt appearance, poor nutritional status, parotid swelling.
• **Viral hepatitis** — needle marks (? IVDU), tattoos
• **Non-alcoholic fatty liver disease** — arcus senilis, xanthelasma, tendon xanthomata, evidence of finger prick (diabetes)
• **Primary Biliary cirrhosis** — Middle aged female, pruritus/scratch marks, xanthelasma
• **PSC** — associated with inflammatory bowel disease; think about it in young, clubbed patient with multiple abdominal scars and stoma
• **Haemochromatosis** — 'bronzed' diabetes (slate grey pigmentation & finger prick marks), scars (venesection scars, liver biopsy, roof top incision fur hemi hepatectomy for HCC, joint replacements)
• **Wilson's disease** — Kayser-Fleischer rings, young patient with movement disorder
• **HCC** — cachexia, tender hepatomegaly
• **CCF/RHF** — raised JVP, enlarged tender liver, peripheral oedema. Alcohol, haemochromatosis & Wilson's disease can cause cardiomyopathy
• **Alpha one antitrypsin deficiency**: evidence of COPD

Signs of Decompensation (ABCDE, the corresponding Child Pugh score elements highlighted)	Features of Portal Hypertension
• Ascites (Albumin, Distention)
• Jaundice (Bilirubin)
• Bruising (Clotting)
• Asterixis (Encephalopathy)
• Altered GCS (Encephalopathy)
• Evidence of portal hypertension	• Splenomegaly (Hypersplenism)
• Caput medusa
• Venous hum

Sample Presentation

Thank you for asking me to examine this patient who was comfortable at rest. He has several stigmata of Chronic Liver Disease. In his hands, there is evidence of clubbing, Dupuytren's contracture, and palmer erythema. On his arms and torso there are numerous spider naevi. He has jaundiced sclerae, and evidence of gynaecomastia. Examination of his abdomen revealed a distended abdomen with evidence of shifting dullness in keeping with ascites. As a result, demonstration of hepatomegaly and splenomegaly was difficult. There was some mild bruising in the flanks. I believe he has decompensated liver disease as evidenced by his ascites and jaundice and evidence of probable coagulopathy with visible bruising. He has no evidence of encephalopathy such as deranged GCS or asterixis.

I would like to suggest alcohol as the most likely aetiology as there is evidence of parotid enlargement. Other differentials to consider include viral hepatitis as he has tattoos on his arms. Autoimmune and metabolic aetiologies cannot be excluded from physical examination and would also need to be considered in the differential by taking a careful history, with attention to past medical history, family history and drug history.

Discussion topics: Differential diagnoses, Investigations, Management (specifically CHILD PUGH Score; Ascites)

Differential Diagnoses

- Alcoholic liver disease
- Viral hepatitis (Hepatitis B, Hepatitis C, Cytomegalovirus, Epstein Barr virus, Yellow fever)
- Non-alcoholic fatty liver disease
- Autoimmune liver disease (Autoimmune hepatitis, Primary biliary cirrhosis, Primary sclerosing cholangitis)
- Metabolic disease (Haemochromatosis, Wilson's Disease, α 1 Antitrypsin deficiency)
- Others: Cardiac (congestive hepatopathy secondary to right heart failure) & Vascular (Budd Chiari or portal vein thromboses) causes are rare.

Causes of hepatomegaly: Mention causes beginning with C first (bold) as they are more common than those beginning with I. Your differential diagnoses should be guided by your clinical findings. At this level, you are not just expected to make a diagnosis of the condition, but also to identify the cause & complications (of disease & treatment) and how the disease has affected your patient's functional capacity.

Non-Tender Hepatomegaly	Tender Hepatomegaly

• **Cirrhosis — alcoholic liver disease**
• Immunological causes —
  Autoimmune liver disease
  Primary sclerosing cholangitis
  Autoimmune hepatitis
• Infiltrative disorders including lymphoproliferative & myeloproliferative disorders, amyloidosis.
	• **Cancer (HCC or secondary)**
	• **Congestive hepatopathy (Right Heart Failure)**
	• Infections (Acute viral hepatitis)

Investigations	Management

• Full blood count
• Coagulation screen
• Liver function tests
• Urea and Electrolytes
• Glucose
• Liver screen:
  ▪ Viral Serology
  ▪ Auto antibodies including AMA (PBC — M2 subtype 95%, PSC) ASMA (AIH & PSC) Anti LKM 1(AIH) ANCA (PSC — 80%)
  ▪ Ferritin, Transferrin saturation (Hereditary haemochromatosis)
  ▪ Caeruloplasmin (Wilson's Disease)
  ▪ Alpha one antitrypsin
  ▪ Alpha feto-protein (HCC)
• Ultrasound abdomen/Fibroscan
• Ascitic tap to rule out SBP (if WBC >250/mm^3)
Serum Ascites: Albumin Gradient ≥11 is suggestive of transudative pathology (Cirrhosis, Cardiac failure, Nephrotic syndrome). Check ascitic fluid amylase if pancreatic pathology suspected.
 	
Further investigations:
Liver biopsy, OGD with or without colonoscopy, Radiological investigations including chest radiography and CT abdomen/pelvis where malignancy is suspected.
	• **Don't forget general measures**
	MDT approach
	Early specialist intervention
	Patient education
	Alcohol withdrawal services referral
	Dietitian input to maintain adequate nutrition.
	Avoid hepatotoxic medications (NSAIDs, Benzodiazepines)
	• **Manage underlying aetiology:**
	Alcohol abstinence
	Steroids for AIH
	Ursodeoxycholic acid for PBC
	Antivirals for Viral Hepatitis
	• **Manage ascites:** Diuretics (First line — Spironolactone up to 400 mg/day and second line — Furosemide up to 160 mg/day), low salt diet (< 5.2 g/day), paracentesis with synthetic plasma expanders, TIPSS (transjugular intrahepatic portosystemic shunt).
	BSG (British Society of Gastroenterology) no longer recommend bed rest & fluid restriction; BSG recommend cautious monitoring of serum Na with advice to withhold diuretics at Na <125 mmol/l and use volume expanders (Please see BSG website).
	• **Manage encephalopathy:** lactulose
	• **Manage portal hypertension/varices:** propranolol, OGD and banding, TIPSS
	• **Consider referral for liver transplant** — Please learn King's College Criteria for referral to liver transplant units.

Managing Spontaneous Bacterial Peritonitis (SBP): Diagnostic paracentesis for all cirrhotic patients admitted to hospital with ascites and those with features of peritoneal infection including the development of encephalopathy, renal impairment, or peripheral leucocytosis without a precipitating factor. Empiric antibiotic therapy with third generation cephalosporins (check local guidelines). Patients with SBP and signs of developing renal impairment should be given albumin at 1.5 g/kg in the first six hours followed by 1 g/kg on day 3. Give prophylaxis with continuous oral Norfloxacin 400 mg/day (or Ciprofloxacin at 500 mg once daily) and refer for liver transplantation if they fulfil relevant criteria following recovery.

Additional Case: Haemochromatosis

Presentation: CLD, Generally unwell, Fatigue, Arthritis, HCC.

Clinical Signs: To be presented as a case of CLD but comment on slate grey pigmentations, hepatomegaly & scars (including venesection scars, liver biopsy, roof top incision fur hemi hepatectomy for HCC, and joint replacements). Also comment on arthropathy and evidence of diabetes (insulin needle marks, fingertip marks from glucose monitoring).

Investigations: As in CLD but workup to include family screening and iron studies. If ferritin and transferrin saturations abnormal to proceed to liver biopsy and genotype analyses. Look for evidence of complications (Cardiomyopathy — echocardiography; Diabetes — OGTT, HbA1c; HCC — alpha fetoprotein, USS liver).

Treatment: Regular venesection, abstinence of alcohol, HCC surveillance and liver transplantation once cirrhosis established. As with all hereditary conditions, do not forget to mention FAMILY SCREENING.

Complications: DM, hypogonadism (usually secondary), testicular atrophy, cardiomyopathy, arthropathy, Hepatocellular carcinoma.

Additional Case: Liver Transplant

Clinical Signs

- Mercedes Benz scar/Modified rooftop incision.
- Evidence of immunomodulatory therapy (please see Case 1: Renal replacement therapy)
- Evidence of underlying disease (please see Case 2: Chronic liver disease)

Sample Presentation

This patient has a transplanted liver as evidenced by a classical Mercedes Benz scar. I would like to present an aetiology of…. (*differentials listed*). There is evidence of immunomodulatory therapy as evidenced by gum hypertrophy (Ciclosporin)/Cushingoid appearance (Steroids)/Tremor (Tacrolimus)/Scars of skin cancer removal (Tacrolimus/Azathioprine). At present, there are no signs of hepatic decompensation suggesting that the transplant is functional.

Common causes of liver transplantation in UK:

- Chronic liver disease
- Acute liver failure (Paracetamol & Viral hepatitis being the most common causes)
- Malignancy (Hepatocellular carcinoma)

Management: MDT approach; Patient education; Treatment of cause; Treat infections & complications; Specialist input; Supportive treatment & follow up.

Problems following transplantation:

- Graft dysfunction
- Acute or chronic rejection
- Recurrence of original disease
- Lymphoproliferative disease
- Infections (CMV, PCP) and Immunosuppressant drug toxicity
- Cancers (skin, haematological) and cardiovascular disease (hypertension, hyperlipidaemia).

Case 3: Splenomegaly

Clinical Examination

Classical Signs	Additional Signs Suggesting Cause
• Spleen enlarged towards right iliac fossa	• CLD with portal hypertension — see Case 2. • Haematological malignancy — Petechiae, purpura, pyrexia, lymphadenopathy, Evidence of bone marrow biopsy — plasters. • Endocarditis — Splinter haemorrhages, Temperature chart, cannula for IV antibiotics; ask for urine dipstick for blood and mention fundoscopy for Roth's Spots. • Felty's syndrome — Rheumatoid hands.

It is important to have a clear set of differential diagnosis and present the case according to the diagnosis it best fits in to as guided by clinical findings.

Sample Presentation 1

The patient is anaemic as evidenced by conjunctival pallor and there are no peripheral stigmata of liver disease. There is a symmetrical deforming arthropathy affecting small joints of both hands with ulnar deviation of the wrists and visible rheumatoid nodules on elbows and multiple joint replacement scars. The spleen is palpable 3 cm below the costal margin with a palpable notch and percussion over Traube's space (left 9th–11th intercostal space) is dull. It moves towards the right iliac fossa with respiration and is not ballotable. I cannot get above the swelling. There is no hepatomegaly, ascites, peripheral oedema or venous hum. There are no signs of hepatic encephalopathy. In absence of signs of portal hypertension and CLD, the most likely diagnosis is Felty's syndrome.

Sample Presentation 2

The patient is anaemic as evidenced by conjunctival pallor. There are excoriation marks suggestive of pruritus. The spleen is palpable 8 cm below the costal margin with a palpable notch and there is dullness to percussion over Traube's space (left 9th–11th intercostal space). There is no hepatomegaly, ascites, peripheral oedema or venous hum. There are no peripheral stigmata of liver disease or connective tissue disease. There are no signs of hepatic encephalopathy. In absence of signs of portal hypertension, liver disease and lymphadenopathy, the most likely diagnosis is myeloproliferative disease.

Note: Dullness to percussion over Traube's space has a 90% sensitivity for splenomegaly.

Discussion topics: Differential diagnoses, Investigations, Management

Differential diagnoses: Mention causes in bold first. Tropical infections are rare in the United Kingdom.

- **Haematological causes: Myeloproliferative and lymphoproliferative disorders, Haemolytic anaemias**
- **CLD with portal hypertension**
- Infections (Spontaneous bacterial endocarditis, Malaria, Kala azar, Hepatitis, HIV)
- Felty's Syndrome (with Rheumatoid arthritis; triad of RA, neutropaenia, splenomegaly)
- Infiltrative disorders (Amyloid/Gaucher's) (unlikely to come up in the exam)

Causes of massive splenomegaly:

- CML
- Myelofibrosis
- Chronic malaria
- Visceral Leishmaniasis.

Investigations

Haematological Cause	Infectious Aetiology	CLD with Portal HTN
• Full blood count • Peripheral blood film • Inflammatory markers including ESR & CRP.	• Full blood count • Peripheral blood film including for malarial parasites	• Full blood count • Coagulation screen • Liver function tests • Urea and Electrolytes • Glucose

• Coagulation profile.
• Serum LDH
• CT for staging.
• Lymph node biopsy
• Bone marrow aspirate
• Genetic tests (BCR-ABL1)
	• Inflammatory markers
	• Viral serology
	• Blood cultures & Echo (SBE)
	• Serology/Bone marrow/Splenic aspirate for amastigotes (Visceral leishmaniasis)
		• Liver screen
		  ➤ Viral Serology
		  ➤ Auto antibodies
		  ➤ Haematinics & Iron Studies
		  ➤ Caeruloplasmin
		  ➤ Alpha one antitrypsin
		  ➤ Alpha fetoprotein
		• Ultrasound abdomen +/− Fibroscan
		• Ascitic tap
		
		Further investigations:
		Liver biopsy, OGD with or without colonoscopy

Treating haematological malignancies:

- **General measures:** MDT approach, Early specialist input, Patient Education, Dietitian input to maintain adequate nutritional intake.
- **Supportive treatment:** Replacement of deficient blood products as per haematology advice. Early treatment of infections.
  - Dysfunctional RBC — Anaemia — Blood transfusion
  - Dysfunctional WBC — Infections — Antibiotics
  - Dysfunctional Platelets — Coagulopathy & bleeding — Platelet transfusion
- **Specific management:** Guided by stage of disease with chemo/radiotherapy and immunotherapy usually in three phases (Remission induction/Remission consolidation/Remission maintenance).
- **Palliative care input:** End stage disease.

Myeloproliferative disorders & their treatment summarised:

Cells	Disease	Treatment
RBC	Polycythaemia rubra vera (JAK2 mutation)	Venesection Hydroxycarbamide Alpha interferon Aspirin
WBC	Chronic myeloid leukaemia (Philadelphia chromosome; translocation of genetic material between chromosome 9 and chromosome 22, and contains a fusion gene called BCR-ABL1; found in 95 %)	Supportive treatment Tyrosine kinase inhibitors
Platelets	Essential thrombocythaemia	Low dose aspirin Hydroxycarbamide (>60 years)
Fibroblasts	Myelofibrosis	Platelet derived growth factor Allogenic bone marrow transplantation

INDEX

Abdominal discomfort, 40–42
Abdominal examination, 197–198
Acromegaly, 84–87
Adrenal insufficiency, 45
Anaemia, 57, 199–200, 210–211
Angina, 37, 138
Ankylosing spondylitis, 70–72
Aortic regurgitation, 71, 139–140
Aortic stenosis, 137–138
Argyll Robertson Pupil, 193
Asbestos related disease, 18, 127
Ascites, 203–204, 206
Asthma (occupational), 50–52
Atrial Fibrillation, 142, 143, 195

Bell's palsy, 198
Beneficence, 3
Breaking bad news, 9–11
Bronchiectasis, 120, 124–125
Bronchogenic carcinoma, 118–120
Bulbar palsy, 155, 172–174

Capacity, 3
Cardiology examination, 133–134
Cerebellar syndrome, 182, 161–162
Charcot Marie Tooth Disease, 166
Chronic liver disease, 47–49, 203–208
Cirrhosis, 203–208
Cranial nerves, 186–190
Crohn's disease, 40–42
Communication, 2–25
Competence, 3, 5–7, 23
Confidentiality, 9–11, 15, 19
Consent, 23
COPD, 130–132
COVID 19, 36
Cushing's Syndrome, 93–96
Cystic fibrosis, 122–125

Demyelination, 161–162, 182–185
Diabetes, 104–109, 163
Diabetic retinopathy, 104–109
Diarrhoea, 40–42
DMARD, 68
Driving restrictions, 14–16
Dysarthria, 155–156, 161–162

Epilepsy, 14, 101–102
Ethics, 2–3

Facial nerve palsy, 190
Friedrich's ataxia, 175
Fundoscopy, 103–112

Gillick competence, 23
Goitre, 88–92
Grave's disease, 88–92
Guillain Barre Syndrome, 164

Haemochromatosis, 207
Headache, 34–35
Hepatomegaly, 205
History taking for PACES, 28–33
Holme's Adie pupil, 192–193
Horner's syndrome, 191
Human Organ Transplant Act, 22
Human Tissue Act (1961), 22
Huntington's Chorea, 25, 160
Hypertensive retinopathy, 110
Hyperthyroidism, 88–92
Hypothyroidism, 88–92

IMCA, 7
Inflammatory bowel disease, 40–42, 54–56
Internuclear ophthalmoplegia, 182–185

Interstitial lung disease, 56, 74, 123, 126–127
Ischaemic heart disease, 16, 37

Jaundice, 197–198, 203–208

Leukaemia, 210–211
Liver function test, 47–48, 206
Liver transplant, 208
Lobectomy, 118–120
Lung transplant, 122
Lymphoma, 210–211

Marcus Gunn Pupil, 186–187
Marfan's Syndrome, 139–140
Mental Capacity Act, 3
Mesothelioma, 18
Mitral regurgitation, 143–145
Mitral stenosis, 141–142
Motor neuron disease, 172–174
Multiple sclerosis, 154, 161–162, 182–185, 186
Myasthenia gravis, 168–170
Myotonic dystrophy, 159–160
Myocardial infarction, 16, 37

Negligence, 19–20
Neurofibromatosis, 98–100
Neurology examination, 151–156

Occupational asthma, 50–52
Optic atrophy, 186–187

Pansystolic murmurs, 143–149
Papilloedema, 110
Paraesthesia, 163–167
Parkinsonism, 157–158

Peripheral neuropathy, 163–167
Pleural effusion, 128–129
Pneumonectomy, 118–120
Pneumonia, 129
Polycystic kidney disease, 201–202
Prosthetic valves, 135–136
Proximal myopathy, 88, 168
Pseudobulbar palsy, 155, 172–174
Psoriatic arthropathy, 54, 63–69
Pulmonary fibrosis, 56, 74, 123, 126–127

Raynaud's, 55, 73–77
Renal transplant, 199–200
Respiratory examination, 115–117
Rheumatoid arthritis, 57–62

Splenomegaly, 209–211
Stroke, 194–195
Syncope, 43–46
Syringomyelia, 178–179
SLE, 78–82
Systemic sclerosis, 73–77

TIA, 194–195
Tremor, 157–158, 161–162
Tricuspid regurgitation, 146–147
Tuberculosis, 120–121
Tuberous sclerosis, 101–102

Ulcerative colitis, 40–42

Ventricular septal defect, 148–149

Wheeze, 50–52, 124, 130–131
Wilson's Disease, 49